CURING
HEPATITIS
C

CURING HEPATITIS C

Current and Future Options for Treatment

Gregory T. Everson, M.D., F.A.C.P

Foreword by Eugene R. Schiff, M.D.

>> hatherleigh

Hatherleigh Press is committed to preserving and protecting the natural resources of the earth. Environmentally responsible and sustainable practices are embraced within the company's mission statement. Hatherleigh Press is a member of the Publishers Earth Alliance, committed to preserving and protecting the natural resources of the planet while developing a sustainable business model for the book publishing industry.

DISCLAIMER
This book does not give legal or medical advice. Always consult your doctor, lawyer, and other professionals. The names of people who contributed anecdotal material have been changed.

The ideas and suggestions contained in this book are not intended as a substitute for consulting with a physician. All matters regarding your health require medical supervision.

Library of Congress Cataloging-in-Publication Data is available.
ISBN: 978-1-57826-425-4

All Hatherleigh Press titles are available for bulk purchase, special promotions, and premiums. For information about reselling and special purchase opportunities, please call 1-800-528-2550 and ask for the Special Sales Manager.

Cover Design by Dede Cummings Designs
Interior Design by Dede Cummings Designs

Printed in the United States

10 9 8 7 6 5 4 3 2 1

))) hatherleigh

www.hatherleighpress.com

CONTENTS

DEDICATION

I dedicate this book to my wife, Linda, and sons, Brad and Todd—you're the greatest!

—*Gregory T. Everson*, M.D., F.A.C.P.

ACKNOWLEDGMENTS

I WANT TO FIRST acknowledge the patients who were evaluated for chronic hepatitis C and were treated in the hepatology clinics and clinical research centers at the University of Colorado-Denver. In particular, I want to thank those patients who contributed their personal stories or remarks—without your input, this book would have been just another "dry" text full of data.

I greatly appreciate and gratefully acknowledge the hard-working, dedicated members of the Liver Team at the University of Colorado-Denver, who are always generous with help and support: Hugo Rosen, M.D., James Burton, M.D., Lisa Forman, M.D., Scott Biggins, M.D., Kiran Bambha, M.D., Sarah Tise, P.A., Lynette Driscoll, P.A., Michelle Miller R.N., Catherine Ray, R.N., B.S.N., M.A., Anne Shaver, R.N., Mindy Stewart, R.N., Wendy Starkey, R.N., Jennifer Rust, R.N., Catherine Behnke, R.N., Andrea Petties, Cheryl Brinton, Igal Kam, M.D., Michael Wachs, M.D., Thomas Bak, M.D., Michael Zimmerman, M.D., Marge Frueh, R.N., Jennifer DeSanto, R.N., Lauri Filar, B.A., Andrea Herman, R.N., Halley Isberg, B.A., Seda Ozdemir, B.A., Shannon Lauriski, B.S., Steve Helmke Ph.D., Michelle Jaramillo, Rita Lerner, Stasia Krajec, Phyllis Titsworth, Tracy Steinberg, R.N., M.S., C.C.T.C, Lana Schoch, R.N., Kathy Orban, R.N., Lauren Myers, R.N., Heather Kappelli, R.N., Michael Talamantes, M.S.S.W., L.C.S.W, the floor and ICU nurses at University of Colorado Hospital, and staff at the General Clinical Research Center and Clinical Translational Research Center at University of Colorado Hospital and the University of Colorado-Denver.

PREFACE

C URING HEPATITIS C: Current and Future Options for Treatment presents an entirely different theme to you, the reader: hepatitis C *can* be cured! Obviously, this book is an offshoot of a previous book, *Living with Hepatitis C: A Survivor's Guide*, authored by Hedy Weinberg and myself through five editions.

Hedy Weinberg and I wrote *Living with Hepatitis C: A Survivor's Guide* for the purpose of providing patients and caregivers with an authoritative, readily available resource. I composed the medical information, and Hedy presented the patient perspective by interviewing many patients with HCV to develop a personal connection for the reader. In this new book, I have focused on issues and questions related to the current new standard of treatment—triple therapy—and other exciting, emerging therapies. As treatment options continue to improve, eradication of HCV infection will become increasingly common; the new paradigm will be living without (not with) hepatitis C. Perhaps I am overly optimistic, but I believe that it is entirely possible that the emerging treatments will be so potent and effective that nearly every patient with chronic hepatitis C may be cured by future antiviral therapies.

The first edition of *Living with Hepatitis C: A Survivor's Guide* was published in 1997. At that time, there was scant information regarding the hepatitis C virus, and the prevailing treatment, interferon monotherapy, was largely ineffective. When the first test for the virus had become available around 1990, newly diagnosed patients asked questions, but, unfortunately, physicians had relatively few answers. As the years went by, our knowledge grew, and so did the task of educating the rapidly growing number of people diagnosed with hepatitis C.

To meet the public's need for information about hepatitis C, I gave lectures to patients and families in Denver, Colorado, and at the University of Colorado's Health Sciences Center. I first met Hedy Weinberg at one of these presentations. After the lecture, Hedy, a hepatitis C patient and writer, approached me and suggested that we turn the lecture series into a guidebook for our patients at the hepatology clinics at the University of Colorado Hospital. What had begun as a simple pamphlet quickly turned into a long-term project, which resulted in the publication of the first edition of *Living with Hepatitis C: A Survivor's Guide.*

Over the next four editions, we wrote and rewrote the text to create an updated, useful guide that would take the patient step-by-step through the process of diagnosis and ongoing care. We anticipated questions, translated medical jargon, and attempted to reduce the fear of the unknown. Therefore, we also presented overviews of emotional, financial, and nutritional issues that accompany this chronic illness. We further added new chapters dealing with liver cancer, co-infection, and children. In the pages of our books, you heard the voices of patients and staff at the University of Colorado Hospital and the University of Colorado's Health Sciences Center, who generously contributed their knowledge and experiences, encouraging us to complete the work.

So, why change? Why not just update *Living with Hepatitis C: A Survivor's Guide* for a sixth edition? There were several reasons to change this focus and produce an entirely new book for patients and families, which you now hold in your hands. First and foremost, treatments for hepatitis C are increasingly effective. Second, patients who had cleared hepatitis C with past treatments have now been followed for more than 10 years and remain free of infection—the word *cure* is becoming part of the lexicon of hepatitis C. Better treatments and the possibility of a cure have persuaded me to take an entirely different point of view; instead of simply surviving with this potentially deadly virus, it is now possible to seek treatment and knowledge to eradicate the infection and live a fuller, longer life. This new book is specifically treatment-oriented. My goals are to familiarize you with descriptions of the current drugs and outcomes, detail the first direct-acting antivirals approved by the FDA (telaprevir and boceprevir), and update you on the results from early-phase clinical trials of new drugs in development.

Another reason to shift focus is authorship. You will note that I am the sole author of this text. Hedy was cured of hepatitis C through treatment with interferon and ribavirin, and her interests, activities, and projects have now carried her in other directions beyond (or beside) the HCV story. I am so pleased that she has been cured, and I wish her all the best in her future endeavors.

Although *Curing Hepatitis C: Current and Future Options for Treatment* is a detailed treatment guide, it does not replace the advice and care of your physician, nor does it give legal advice. Instead, it is designed solely to educate patients and their families about hepatitis C treatments. Consult appropriate specialists, and always work closely with your doctor when making medical decisions.

FOREWORD

THERE HAVE BEEN dramatic advances in our understanding of hepatitis C in recent years and the latest treatments have proven to be highly effective with tolerable side effects. However, many patients wonder whether these new treatments are contraindicated due to severity of disease and drug-drug interactions. In addition, various other questions have arisen among patients regarding new and upcoming treatments. *Curing Hepatitis C: Current and Future Options for Treatment* has come at an optimal time and is sure to help answer many of these questions.

We are quickly approaching the availability of interferon-free direct antiviral regimens that will cure the majority of patients with hepatitis C, regardless of previous treatment experience. In addition, major efforts towards routine HCV screening of people, particularly between the ages of 45 or 65, are underway. In contrast to the management of hepatitis C patients in the recent past, newly diagnosed patients will now be treated shortly after diagnosis because of the high cure rates with much more tolerable treatment regimens. All of these recent advancements mean that hepatitis C treatment is progressing towards a "test, treat, and *cure*" approach.

Curing Hepatitis C is written in a very practical and understandable style by an outstanding world-renowned author with extensive hands-on experience. Updated diagnostic, epidemiologic, serologic, and current (as well as future) therapeutic aspects are discussed in straightforward language. In short, this book will serve as an excellent resource to anyone afflicted with hepatitis C.

EUGENE R. SCHIFF, M.D.

1

THE BASICS OF HEPATITIS C
An Introduction

I went to my doctor for a regular checkup, not because I felt sick (although I was fatigued). The blood tests showed that my liver enzymes were just slightly abnormal—the tests were repeated and still abnormal. Then my doctor did more tests and found that I tested positive for an antibody against hepatitis C. Next thing you know, I had a liver biopsy.

The results indicated chronic hepatitis C. My stomach clenched, and I felt a cold rush of fear—I didn't know what hepatitis C was or what to expect.

— Rhonda

THE INFORMATION in this chapter has been extracted, updated, and modified from chapters 1 and 3 of the fifth edition of *Living with Hepatitis C: A Survivor's Guide*. If you want additional, more detailed information, please refer to the original chapters in the fifth edition of *Living with Hepatitis C*.

UNDERSTANDING HEPATITIS C

To help you understand hepatitis C, I will define three terms:

1. hepatitis
2. virus
3. hepatitis C virus (HCV)

What Is Hepatitis? Hepatitis simply means inflammation of the liver. Hepatitis is caused not only by the hepatitis C virus (HCV), but also by other viruses, alcohol, medications, drugs, or toxins.

Unfortunately, the public hears so many stories of celebrities who have injured their livers with substance abuse that they tend to lump all forms of liver disease together. As anyone with hepatitis C can tell you, it is not uncommon (although extremely unfair) to be labeled an alcoholic, even if you have never taken a drink.

> *When I finally tell someone I have hepatitis C, the atmosphere changes. I've had people give me this airbrush handshake, because they don't want to touch me. Or, they'll say, "Isn't that what that baseball star had? Didn't he drink himself to death?" Suddenly, there's this invisible wall.*
>
> *— Sara*

During the past 50 years, scientists have discovered many viruses that cause disease; not just the hepatitis viruses, but others like HIV. Each virus has its own way of infecting people, but it is hard for the public to see the differences.

> *It's an awkward moment when you let friends know you have this disease. They don't know what to say, and most of what they know about viruses has to do with AIDS, so you get a lot of weird stares and silences. You can see the stereotypes running through their heads. I'm so tired of explaining that the virus is almost never passed sexually, that it's a blood-to-blood thing.*
>
> *— Bob*

What Is a Virus? The term "virus" evokes fear in people—fear of the unknown, the invisible. Viruses are not visible to the human eye or even under a microscope. You need a special tool, such as an electron microscope, to see them. Despite their small size, viruses carry genetic material with enough punch to injure our organs and bodies, and even cause death[1].

Viruses are as old as humankind, possibly older. Archeologists have unearthed an Egyptian mummy that bears pockmarks, evidence of the smallpox virus from thousands of years ago. Among other diseases, viruses cause polio, mononucleosis, rabies, herpes, yellow fever, influenza, measles, rubella, chickenpox, mumps, and the common cold—as well as new plagues, such as ebola and AIDS.

"A virus," said Nobel Laureate Sir Peter Medawar, "is a piece of bad news wrapped in protein."[2]—and that about sums it up. The "bad news" of a virus is its code, which is its center of nucleic acid (the viral genes) —either ribonucleic acid (RNA) or deoxyribonucleic acid (DNA). Viruses also have "coats," which are made of specific proteins unique to the virus.

When a virus's coat attaches to a cell in the body, the virus's genes enter the cell. It orders the cell to stop its own work and to make more viruses, instead. In time, the virus multiplies to infect other cells.

Alerted to danger, the body's immune system sends out antibodies (special types of proteins) to stick to the invading virus and neutralize it. Viruses, however, are able to change and mutate to evade these antibodies.

The hepatitis C virus is particularly good at mutating, which makes it difficult for scientists to create a vaccine. It has been hard to hit this moving target.

What Is the Hepatitis C Virus? The hepatitis C virus (HCV), also known as hepacivirus, is a single-stranded ribonucleic acid (RNA) virus, and is a type of flavivirus, a family of viruses that produce yellow fever, dengue, and Japanese encephalitis[3]. Four million Americans and over 160 million persons worldwide are infected with HCV (Figure 1A).

FIGURE I A: GLOBAL PREVALENCE OF HEPATITIS C

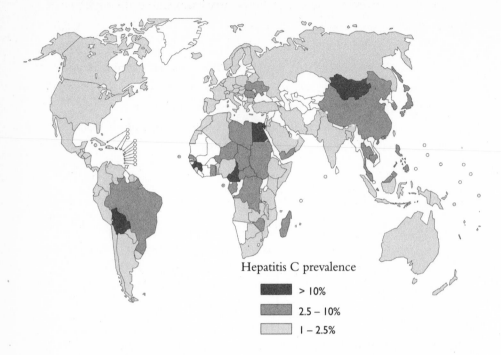

Hepatitis C prevalence

■ > 10%
■ 2.5 – 10%
□ 1 – 2.5%

FIGURE I A: The worldwide distribution of hepatitis C according to 2001 statistics from the World Health Organization is shown. The dark shaded areas indicate regions of the world with the highest prevalence of hepatitis C.

Genotypes of HCV. To complicate the hepatitis C picture even more, at least six distinct genetic strains (or genotypes) of HCV have been identified[4]. The HCV genotypes are designated as genotypes 1 through 6[5]. The most common genotype in the United States and Europe is HCV genotype 1, accounting for nearly 75 percent of cases. HCV genotype 3 is common in Australia, HCV genotype 4 predominates in the Middle East, HCV genotype 5 is common in Indonesia and South Africa, and HCV genotype 6 is common in Southeast Asia[6].

HCV RNA. How do you know if you are infected with HCV? The only sure way to tell is to test for HCV by measuring HCV RNA in your blood. If HCV RNA is positive, then you are infected with HCV. If HCV RNA is undetectable, then you are not infected with HCV.

Hepatitis C is transmitted by blood, like hepatitis B. Unlike hepatitis B and HIV, however, it seems to be poorly transmitted through sexual contact[7].

> We've been married 15 years. I told my wife—and the doctor told my wife—that she doesn't have hepatitis C after sleeping with me all these years, and that it would be extremely rare to get it from sex.
>
> We could use protection if that would help her feel safer—but it's pretty lonely. She doesn't even hug me anymore.
>
> — Ralph

You may not be able to recall when you were initially infected with the hepatitis C virus. Lack of symptoms is common during the initial acute infection. Symptoms, when they occur, are often mild. In fact, if you had symptoms from acute hepatitis C, you might have interpreted them as a case of the flu.

Natural History. Twenty-five to 45 percent of patients clear HCV after acute infection. In the follow-up of these cases, the antibody against HCV (HCV-Ab) is positive, but HCV RNA is undetectable. The ability to clear HCV spontaneously, without treatment, depends upon the genetics of a person's interferon responsiveness. The key determinant is a special type of genetic factor called the IL28b polymorphism, which defines your body's responsiveness to interferon. Persons with the CC genotype of the IL28b polymorphism are those most likely to clear HCV spontaneously[8].

Most patients do not clear HCV after acute infection, but rather, develop a long-term (chronic) infection, and have persistently positive tests for HCV RNA. During chronic infection, you may have no symptoms or very mild symptoms (most commonly fatigue). Liver enzymes may be normal or only slightly abnormal. Two chronically infected persons may have identical symptoms and liver enzyme tests, but very different results from a biopsy, from mild, benign changes to advanced injury and even cirrhosis[9].

Hepatitis C typically progresses slowly: only one in four patients with chronic hepatitis C will progress to cirrhosis in the course of a lifetime. Those that do progress, however, may face complications of cirrhosis (such as ascites, jaundice, bleeding, and spells of mental confusion), may need liver transplantation, or may die from liver disease.

> *Way back in the 90s, when I was first diagnosed . . . I had this for a long time and did not know . . . . the doctor who diagnosed me thought the hepatitis C would move fast. He told me I would be dead in five years! I said to myself, "I have to make money for my family." That's why I began my business. Later, I got a second opinion, and was reassured that I'd be around for awhile. Not only did I see my kids through college, but now I even have an eight-month-old grandson!*
>
> — *Mark*

If you have chronic hepatitis C, there is actually some very good news! Many treatments are available or under study for the treatment of chronic hepatitis C[10]. You may be a candidate for one of these treatments. The new standard of care for patients infected with HCV genotype 1 is triple therapy, which is discussed in detail in chapters 4 and 5[11]. The previous standard of care for all HCV genotypes, peginterferon plus ribavirin (see chapter 3), is still the current standard therapy for non-1 HCV genotypes. Several new drugs, which inhibit key viral pathways or modify host responses, may have activity against all HCV genotypes and are discussed in some detail in chapter 6.

When you have chronic hepatitis C, you should consider evaluation for treatment. Why? If left untreated, hepatitis C can progress, leading to liver failure and liver cancer, and can possibly even require liver transplantation. Today, hepatitis C is the leading indicator for liver transplantation. Nearly half of the patients on liver transplant waiting lists have hepatitis C[12]. Effective treatment, however, can cure you of hepatitis C, and halt the progression of your liver disease.

TRANSMISSION OF HCV
Intravenous Drug Abuse

What is the most direct way to get hepatitis C? Inoculate the virus from infected blood into your own bloodstream. That is why one of the most common risk factors is a history of using illicit intravenous drugs[13, 14]. Many drug addicts share needles. Because of this, they spread hepatitis among themselves and maintain a pool of infected people. Studies suggest that up to 75 percent of current or past users of intravenous drugs may have hepatitis C.

Although heavy drug abusers may be at greatest risk, many people who have hepatitis C report only rare experimentation with drugs in the distant past. Unfortunately, the wise decision to stop taking drugs does not erase the risk from prior use.

"I don't know how I could get hepatitis C from sharing needles. I was always so careful about cleaning them," patients often say. Yet to understand how contamination occurs, you have to appreciate how concentrated the virus is in the blood of infected patients.

The average patient with chronic hepatitis C has a blood concentration of the virus of over a million particles per milliliter of whole blood. That is equivalent to 2,000 particles of virus in the amount of blood that would sit on the head of a small stickpin. With this concentration, it is easy to see how wiping or rinsing a needle with water or salt solutions would not remove all the virus particles. Indeed, a large amount of virus may still remain on the needle.

A concentrated solution of hydrogen peroxide will kill or inactivate the virus, and cleaning needles with this solution may reduce the risk of transmission. Nonetheless, it will not protect you if cleaning is superficial (for example, as a quick rinse), or if the internal chamber of the needle is not irrigated, and the syringe and all its external and internal parts are not cleansed. Some people rely on others to clean a syringe, and do not realize that it has not been done thoroughly.

Intranasal Use of Cocaine

Cocaine causes constriction of the blood vessels in the mucous membrane of the nose, leading to disruption of the lining and ulceration. A well-known consequence of chronic cocaine use is damage to the nasal septum, leaving a hole in the cartilage that separates the two nostrils. Sharing straws during cocaine use, therefore, can lead to blood-to-blood transmission of hepatitis C. A recent epidemiological study for risk factors for hepatitis C found an increased prevalence of hepatitis C with patients who were regular users of cocaine[15].

Transfusion of Blood or Blood Products

I'd never been sick a day in my life. Then in 1974, I had a car crash, and received multiple blood transfusions. After the accident, things were never the same. I used to play ball, but heck—it got to where I was always so tired, I could barely go to the games. Forget playing in them.

— Terry

In the past, the nation's blood supply was contaminated with HCV. If you have received blood products prior to 1992, you are at risk of currently being infected with HCV.

Since 1992, testing for HCV in blood donors has been highly sensitive and specific; screening of blood donors with these tests has virtually eliminated the risk of transmission via this route. Statisticians estimate the current risk of transmission as extremely low, but there is no such thing as zero risk[16, 17].

Needle-Stick Accidents

Healthcare workers face an occupational hazard: needle-stick accidents. Because many hospitalized patients and people who frequent emergency rooms have hepatitis, medical personnel run high risks if they accidentally get stuck with an infected needle, which can easily pierce latex or protective gloves.

In one study of an inner city emergency room at Johns Hopkins Hospital in Baltimore, Maryland, 24 percent of 2,523 patients over age 15 were infected with at least one of three viruses: HIV (6 percent), hepatitis B (5 percent), or hepatitis C (18 percent). Eighty-three percent of the intravenous drug users, 21 percent of the people who had transfusions, and 21 percent of the homosexual male patients had hepatitis C. Of all the patients who were bleeding and who had invasive procedures performed, 30 percent had at least one virus[18].

The good news is safe needle technology has reduced the risk of transmission via needle-stick accidents (see the World Health Organization for a description of Safe Injection Global Network [SIGN])[19].

Tattooing and Body Piercing

Tattooing and body piercing are ancient rites in many cultures. In this country, we are witnessing a recent surge of interest in "body art." The practice of tattooing is particularly common in the military and among gang members and prisoners. It is also becoming an accepted cosmetic practice[20].

Celebrities and athletes have popularized the trend. Unfortunately, even the most benign-appearing tattoo may have its dark side (Figure 1B). Viral hepatitis (mainly hepatitis B) is the best-documented infection transmitted by tattoos, but you can also acquire HCV from tattooing.

FIGURE 1B: HEPATITIS C PATIENT WITH TATTOO

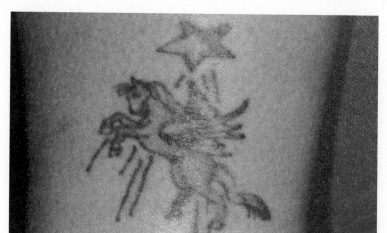

FIGURE 1B: This seemingly innocuous tattoo may have been a source of transmission of hepatitis C to this patient.

Here's a switch: I'm a tattoo artist, and, last year, I found out I have hepatitis C. I have antibodies to hepatitis B, too. My joints hurt so much I can't work. I feel like I'm sliding down the evolutionary scale, because I can't move my opposable thumbs.

I'm sure I got hepatitis from a needle-stick. Fifteen years ago, who wore gloves?

— Peter

Nine percent of males and 1 percent of females in the United States get tattoos, with peak ages between 14 and 22. Furthermore, tattoos are common in certain groups at high risk for hepatitis C and other viral infections: intravenous drug abusers, gang members, prostitutes, and prisoners[21, 22].

This flag on my arm—I was young and in the navy. What did I know? Now, I'm told that there are certified tattoo artists, and if you go to someone reputable, everything is sterilized.

Well, too late for me. It wasn't like that in Hong Kong.

—Jerry

Tattooing involves shaving the skin, placing ink on it, and then pushing the ink through the skin with a needle gun. A small amount of bleeding is common. The problem is sterilization techniques vary, and home-tattooing kits may contain inadequate methods for sterilization. Other problems encountered with tattoo techniques include lack of disposable needles and repeated insertion of tattoo needles into potentially contaminated ink, which is then re-used on other clients.

Body piercing of the earlobes, nose, lips, and other areas also breaks the skin. Therefore, the principles and risk of transmission of hepatitis C are the same as in tattooing. *(Resource: The Alliance for Professional Tattooists (APT) has developed a set of infection control guidelines in association with the FDA for its members. For a copy of "Basic Guidelines for Getting a Tattoo," email info@safetattoos.com or access their website: www.safetattoos.com/faq.htm.)*

Sharing Sharp Instruments

Family and friends who live with hepatitis C patients do not appear to have an increased risk of getting the virus. Nonetheless, you should take care to prevent your blood, which contains hepatitis C, from inoculating another person accidentally.

> *Yesterday, I found my oldest son, a teenager, standing in front of the bathroom mirror and trying to shave for the first time. I got so scared. My husband has hepatitis C.*
>
> *Why didn't we see how fast our son was growing? Why didn't we warn him not to borrow his dad's razor?*
>
> *— Jan*

Talk to family members and explain why it is important to avoid sharing razor blades, nail clippers, scissors, and toothbrushes. These measures are just good hygiene; it is also sensible to bandage any cuts or abrasions, and to safely dispose of menstrual pads and tampons.

Birth and Delivery

If you have hepatitis C, and you are pregnant or planning a family, of course, you are concerned about giving birth to a healthy baby. The period of risk is during delivery, when the mother's and baby's blood may become intermixed. Mothers with hepatitis C, even if otherwise healthy, can transmit the virus to their newborns. The chance of transmitting hepatitis C from mother to baby at the time of delivery is approximately 6 percent. In contrast, mothers with HIV who are also infected with hepatitis C may transmit hepatitis C to their babies 15 percent or more of the time[23].

Mothers with hepatitis C often ask whether they can transmit the virus to their baby through breastfeeding. Current studies do not allow us to draw a definite conclusion. Existing information suggests, however, that hepatitis C is rarely—if ever—transmitted to an infant through breast milk. Even though hepatitis C may be detected in breast milk, it is likely that the baby's digestive juices and enzymes would destroy the virus.

Sexual Transmission

This is one of the most sensitive and troubling topics for patients. The risk of getting hepatitis C through sexual contact is minimal, but some spouses are wary. Trust dissolves, the gap widens, and the couple can end up in divorce court.

It is just as hard for patients who are single. How do you start an intimate relationship without being honest about hepatitis C? How will the other person react?

> *I'm single, and I'm not the smoothest, slickest character around. It's always been hard for me to meet women. Now, I have to tell them I have hepatitis C. When should I tell them? Will they want to have anything to do with me?*
>
> *— Russ*

> *I'm feeling low, depressed. I was dating this guy, and the relationship was going well. It felt right. Then he broke up with me two days ago. I'm trying not to be paranoid—I mean it could have happened anyway—but he broke up with me a week after I told him I had hepatitis C.*
>
> *— Nancy*

Perhaps some solid information will help you come to grips with this issue. Compared to hepatitis B, hepatitis C circulates in your blood at relatively low levels. It is either not detected or is found in low concentrations in body fluids, such as saliva, urine, feces, semen, or vaginal secretions.

The vast majority of sexual partners of patients with hepatitis C test negative for hepatitis C[7, 24, 25, 26]. When a sexual partner does test positive, in most cases, this partner has had other risk factors for acquiring hepatitis C, such as intravenous drug use or exposure to blood or blood products. In studies of heterosexual couples without other risk factors, sexual transmission of hepatitis C is extremely rare: one estimate placed the risk at one chance in ten million sexual exposures[7]. In contrast, epidemiological studies suggest that, in patients with hepatitis C who do not have specific risk factors (such as blood transfusion or tattoos), there is a higher likelihood that those HCV patients would report having a past heterosexual partner with HCV. Overall, the data suggest that heterosexual transmission of hepatitis C is rare in a stable, single-partner relationship.

Sally's diagnosis shocked us. We were completely naive. She worried about giving me hepatitis C, until we learned more and got a pretty good handle on it.

We've been cautious, but it's not like I'm terrified to go near her. We've been together six years, and I saw no reason to treat her differently or to change our behavior, because I was already exposed.

Sally felt dirty. I did everything I could to diffuse that. It didn't affect the way I felt about her. I kissed her the day before the diagnosis, so why not kiss her the day after?

— Ken

My husband got completely paranoid. When I first found out I had hepatitis C, I wanted him to say, "We'll get through this together," but he didn't. He was really nice for a week; then he started getting hostile. He couldn't handle it. I think a big part of it was that we were getting conflicting information about whether or not you can transmit the virus sexually.

We were having troubles before, and I guess the added strain was too much. During my fifth month of interferon, he left me and our three-year-old daughter.

— Danielle

Sexual transmission of hepatitis C may be more frequent in men who have sex with men or in highly promiscuous heterosexuals[25, 26]. Some sexual practices are more traumatic to body tissues. For example, anal intercourse may disrupt the lining of the rectum and allow blood containing hepatitis C to enter the blood of a sexual partner.

Organ Transplantation

Can a person get hepatitis C from a transplanted organ? Yes, if the donor is actively infected with HCV, the virus will infect the recipient of the donor organ. Several studies have addressed this issue.

In one study, 28 percent of patients who had received organs from donors with hepatitis C developed clinical evidence of liver disease during a follow-up period ranging from three months to six-and-a-half years. In a second study, all the recipients who did not have hepatitis C before the transplant, and who had received an organ from a hepatitis C donor, developed hepatitis C after the transplant[27, 28, 29, 30, 31]. Current organ procurement systems test all donors for hepatitis C to avoid transmission of hepatitis C to a susceptible individual.

Can you, as a hepatitis C patient, donate an organ for transplantation? Yes, but your organs would be allocated preferentially to recipients already infected with hepatitis C. So, even though you have hepatitis C, you may still be able to donate your organs for transplant. The organs most commonly used are the kidney and liver, but only if the liver shows no active disease or scarring.

HOW CAN I AVOID INFECTING OTHERS?

My patients often inquire about protecting friends and family from the virus. Here are some common questions people ask:

Is It Okay To Kiss and Hug My Kids? Yes, you can kiss and hug your children, and they can kiss and hug you back. There is no data to suggest that you could infect your children by these actions.

Should I Have Members of My Family Tested for Hepatitis C? The risk of transmission through casual contact between you and other family members, including your spouse, is very low. In general, if the only contact is casual, testing of family members is not necessary.

Transmission via sexual contact is also unlikely in monogamous or single-partner heterosexual relationships. Nonetheless, transmission may occur, and testing may be needed. Clearly, if your spouse or partner has elevated liver enzyme tests, then they should be tested for hepatitis C. All children of infected mothers should be tested. If family members had any blood-to-blood contact, they should also be tested.

Can I Cook for My Family? What If I Cut Myself While I'm Preparing Food? Certainly, you can cook for your family. Even if you cut yourself and get blood in the food, it is unlikely that anyone eating the food will get hepatitis C. The enzymes in the digestive tract will destroy or inactivate the virus.

What If My Child or Friend Eats Food Off My Plate or Uses My Fork? You do not transmit hepatitis C by sharing drinks or food. Hepatitis C is transmitted by contaminated blood entering your bloodstream, not your stomach.

In some Asian cultures, caregivers pre-chew food for babies. It is hypothetically possible to transmit hepatitis C through saliva if the chewer and baby have mouth sores or bloody gums. Sharing of toothbrushes and anything else that might come in contact with blood or body fluids can also expose people to the same hypothetical risks. Even though these are not common or likely infection routes, it makes good common sense to avoid such behaviors for hygienic reasons.

My Teenager Borrowed My Manicure Scissors. Is That a Problem? I recommend that you avoid sharing sharp instruments. There is a possibility that if your teenager cut herself on your scissors, she could inoculate herself with blood you might have left on the scissors. It is best to avoid sharing all sharp instruments, such as nail clippers and razor blades.

We've Been Married for 15 Years. Is It Safe To Have Sex? The existing information indicates that sexual transmission between individuals in a stable, single-partner, monogamous relationship rarely—if ever—occurs. People involved in a stable relationship do not need to alter their sexual practices.

I'm Single. What Should I Tell My Dates? If you are heterosexual and involved with one partner, my sense is sexual transmission is so low that it may not be an issue. On the other hand, you have a trust issue that you have to resolve; that may require disclosing your hepatitis C infection. Place the disclosure in the context of knowing that your hepatitis C infection need not fracture or destroy an otherwise promising relationship. Infected persons may provide additional protection for their partners by using latex condoms in conjunction with other barrier methods.

What About French Kissing? Oral Sex? The details of these types of sexual activity have not been scientifically investigated. If blood barriers (lining of the mouth, lining of the genitalia) are breached, then blood-to-blood transmission may occur.

Should I Always Use Condoms? Latex condoms and safe sex practices are especially suggested for individuals who have multiple sex partners.

Can I Have a Baby? Nurse My Baby? Yes. Mothers who ask these questions are worried about transmitting hepatitis C to their infants. First, the risk of transmission appears to be limited to the time of delivery, when the blood of the mother and infant may become intermixed. Approximately 6 percent of babies born of mothers with hepatitis C develop the infection.

As stated earlier, a newborn swallowing mother's milk is not likely to become infected with HCV. Always discuss these decisions with your pediatrician or care provider.

How Do I Clean Up a Blood Spill? If you have gloves available, use them. If not, take precautions to prevent contact of the blood with your skin or any cuts, abrasions, sores, or wounds on your skin. Take a rag or paper cloth and wipe the spill. If household bleach is available, use diluted bleach at the site of the spill. Dispose of the rag or paper in a plastic bag, and throw it in the garbage. Wash your hands afterward. The term "universal precautions" when dealing with potentially infectious matter means to wear gloves, avoid exposure to infection, and wash your hands.

Is It Necessary To Tell Healthcare Providers, Like My Dentist, That I Have Hepatitis C? Yes. In my opinion, patients should inform dentists and other healthcare professionals who need to perform invasive procedures or operations.

Can I Be an Organ Donor? Yes. Organs from donors infected with hepatitis C virus can be used, usually for recipients who already have hepatitis C.

We learn geology the morning after the earthquake.

— *Emerson*

The beginning of wisdom is to call things by their right names.

— *Chinese proverb*

2

DIAGNOSING HEPATITIS C AND TESTING YOUR LIVER

Antibodies, HCV RNA, HCV Genotypes,
IL28b Genotypes, Liver Biopsies,
Radiologic Imaging, and Blood Tests

Who ever heard of this complicated stuff before hepatitis C? At first, I kept track of my liver enzymes religiously, writing each ALT and AST score on a yellow legal pad. I ignored the other test results!

Now, I understand that the other lab results inform me more about the health of my liver—how it is functioning. Now, when I look at my lab results, it is like looking into my liver without a microscope. I always ask for a copy of my test results, and I keep my own file of test results. In some way, by tracking the numbers, I feel as if I'm doing all that I can on my end!

— Brian

THIS CHAPTER answers questions regarding the tests used to diagnosis hepatitis C and the tests used for assessing your liver disease. If you want additional information regarding tests for hepatitis C and your liver, please refer to chapters 2 and 4 in the fifth edition of *Living with Hepatitis C: A Survivor's Guide*.

DIAGNOSING HEPATITIS C

Essentially, two tests are used:

- An antibody test, HCV-Ab
- A gene test of the virus, HCV RNA

HCV-Ab. A few months after the discovery of hepatitis C in 1989, an antibody specific for infection with HCV (HCV-Ab) became available[1, 3]. Current antibody tests are more sensitive and specific. You may wonder, "Can my diagnosis be wrong?" With current antibody testing, there are so few false positives that a positive HCV-Ab test means one of the following:

- You have an ongoing infection with hepatitis C.
- You have been exposed to hepatitis C, but are not currently infected. (Some lucky people do fight off HCV on their own (as many as 15 to 45 percent; others may respond to interferon and clear the virus.)
- Your newborn was tested, and the HCV-Ab from your bloodstream was passed through the placenta into your newborn's blood stream. The passage of the HCV-Ab from mother to fetus or newborn does not necessarily imply passage of the hepatitis C virus. If only the antibody is transferred, then HCV-Ab usually clears from the baby's blood within six to 12 months. If the hepatitis C virus is transferred, then the baby is infected. In the case of infection, the baby's blood will test positive for both HCV-Ab and HCV RNA.

I found out I had hepatitis C when I donated blood and got a letter from the blood bank. What a shock! I didn't go to a doctor right away, because I had recently changed jobs, and I was waiting for my new insurance papers to arrive. So, I joined a support group to find out what the heck I had.

They were all talking about a test that measured the amount of virus in your blood: HCV RNA. I had the test done, and it came back negative — zero— nothing. Do I have hepatitis C or not?

— Karen

HCV-RNA Assays. Karen tested positive for hepatitis C antibodies. Yet when she took a test that directly measured the virus in her blood, called the HCV-RNA assay, she tested negative. Does she have hepatitis C or not? Today's HCV RNA tests are very sensitive and specific. Karen had an undetectable HCV RNA, which indicates that she was not actively infected[32].

The first time I had an HCV RNA test, the results were mathematical gobbledygook: 5.5 x 10^6 IU per milliliter of blood. What does that mean? Is that high? Low?

I wanted to hear that I had a low level of virus. For days, I was quietly depressed. Many months later, I had another PCR. I was prepared to hear I had the same or higher results. To my surprise, the viral count was down, way down. I was glad, but it also made me begin to accept how little control I have over this virus.

— Hedy

What do the numbers mean? What is high, and what is low? HCV RNA less than 800,000 IU/mL is low. An HCV RNA greater than 800,000 IU/mL is considered high. The level of HCV RNA fluctuates as much as ten- to one hundred-fold, without any treatment or intervention. The level of HCV RNA is useful for tracking response to treatment, but, otherwise, does not predict the severity of liver disease or risk for disease progression.

Genotypes. After you have gone through the tests that indicate you are infected with hepatitis C, the next step is to determine which genotype of hepatitis C that you have[5]. The hepatitis C virus is really a whole family of viruses with six major genotypes. In the United States, genotype 1 infection accounts for 70 to 75 percent of cases. Different genotypes are more common elsewhere in the world (see chapter 1).

Why is determination of HCV genotype so important? We have learned that the genotypes respond differently to various types of therapy. For example, HCV genotype 1 is relatively resistant to peginterferon/ribavirin, but HCV genotypes 2 and 3 are much more sensitive to this treatment. HCV genotypes do not predict the severity of liver disease or risk for disease progression; rather, they are used mainly to guide which type and duration of treatment may be best for you:

- Genotype 1
    Triple Therapy (see chapters 4 and 5)
- Genotype 2 or 3
    Peginterferon/Ribavirin, 24 weeks (see chapter 3)
- Genotype 4, 5, or 6
    Peginterferon/Ribavirin, 48 weeks (see chapter 3)

Subtypes of HCV Genotypes. There are also two main subtypes of HCV genotype 1, 1a and 1b, which may also affect your treatment options [4]. In the past, when using peginterferon/ribavirin, we did not detect much difference in rates of SVR between HCV subtypes 1a versus 1b (SVR refers to viral clearance, and is defined as undetectable HCV RNA at six months or more post-treatment). Now that we are using new direct-acting antivirals (medicines that act like antibiotics against HCV), however, the response of 1a may be different than 1b. HCV genotype 1a may have a slightly lower rate of SVR and higher rate of emergence of resistant viral variants (see chapters 5 and 6 for more information on viral variants and resistance). Patients infected with HCV genotype 1b may have a higher rate of SVR, less risk for the emergence of resistant viral variants, and a greater likelihood to be cured with interferon-free, ribavirin-free treatment regimens (see chapter 6).

TESTING YOUR LIVER
Liver Imaging

Ultrasounds and CT (computed tomography) scans are the most common non-invasive imaging tests for assessing your liver. MRI (magnetic resonance imaging) is typically used to confirm or further define specific

imaging features found by prior ultrasonography or CT. The main use of
these imaging studies in patients with chronic hepatitis C is to evaluate
for liver tumors, liver cancer (also called hepatoma or hepatocellular
carcinoma), or abnormalities of the blood vessels[33].

Ultrasonography (US or Ultrasound). An ultrasonography is a safe
and painless way to investigate the size, structure, and vascular (blood)
supply of the liver. Due to cost considerations, it is the preferred radiologic technique when screening for liver tumors.

In addition, an ultrasonography may be useful during procedures.
For example, your physician may order an ultrasound to pinpoint the
liver's location just before a biopsy.

Computed Tomography (CT) Scan. Unlike an ultrasound, a computed tomography (CT) scan uses a highly sophisticated x-ray machine
to scan the internal organs with minimal radiation. CT scans are used to
confirm the findings of an ultrasound and to get a clearer view, because,
unlike ultrasounds, CT scans are not blocked by air in the bowel. The scans
are also more standardized and much less dependent on the expertise of
the technician performing the test. CT scans help to define the size and
texture of the liver, and can detect an early liver tumor (Figure 2A).

FIGURE 2A: CT SCAN OF HEPATOCELLULAR CARCINOMA (LIVER CANCER)

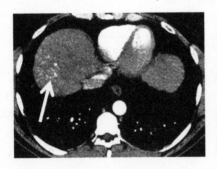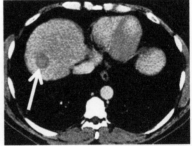

FIGURE 2A: CT (computed tomography) scan of the liver in a patient with
cirrhosis from chronic hepatitis C, demonstrating a 2.7 cm diameter hepatocellular
carcinoma (liver cancer).

Magnetic Resonance Imaging (MRI). Unlike ultrasounds and CT scans, an MRI measures special signals from the body's water molecules or administered test compounds. Images are created from these signals. Magnetic resonance imaging has many applications, and is often used to confirm or delineate abnormalities found on an ultrasonography or CT scan.

Liver Biopsy

Although the word "biopsy" creates anxiety, a biopsy is useful in defining your disease by estimation of the amount of inflammation and fibrosis of the liver[34].

Biopsy Procedure. Liver biopsy is an outpatient procedure, and the biopsy itself takes only a few seconds. In fact, you will spend most of your time getting ready for the biopsy. Liver biopsy is invasive and carries risk (albeit small), so you will be asked to sign an informed consent form.

Your physician first examines you carefully, and often uses an ultra-sound to decide exactly where to place the biopsy needle. The skin is then cleansed with iodine or an antiseptic solution. A local anesthetic is injected underneath the skin and into the tissues where the biopsy needle is to be placed (similar to what is done at the dentist). Some doctors also prescribe intravenous medications to lessen the anxiety and discomfort.

After the biopsy is taken, you will stay in the procedure area for two to four hours for observation. If you are stable with no symptoms, you will be discharged. Otherwise, you may be admitted to the hospital for observation.

After performing biopsies on thousands of patients, I have seen very few complications. Reported rates of complications vary from one in 100 to one in 1,000 cases. In rare cases, the biopsy needle may pierce another organ, such as the bowel, gallbladder, kidney, or lung. Death occurs very rarely, in less than one in 1,000 cases.

Bleeding from the surface of the liver is the most common complication. If bleeding occurs, you may require transfusions or even an operation.

Interpreting Biopsy Results. Your doctor will tell you the results of your biopsy in terms of grades of inflammation and stages of fibrosis. The stage of fibrosis correlates best with liver function and risk for clinical complications[35]. There are four histologic stages of fibrosis due to hepatitis C:

- **Stage I** has minimal scarring (minimal fibrosis).
- **Stage II** features early scarring (fibrosis) in one zone (portal).
- **Stage III** shows bridging of the fibrosis between adjacent portal zones.
- **Stage IV** is cirrhosis (advanced scarring with loss of normal liver architecture).

Liver Blood Tests

Life with hepatitis C means lots of blood tests to monitor your condition. Have you ever wondered what the numbers really mean? Read the next few pages to review and understand the six basic blood tests:

- Enzymes
- Bilirubin
- Albumin
- Prothrombin time (INR)
- Platelet count
- MELD score

Who ever heard of this complicated stuff before hepatitis C? At first, I kept track of my liver enzymes religiously, writing each ALT and AST score on a yellow legal pad. I ignored the other numbers on the lab report.

Now, I understand that the other function tests let me know how my liver is coping with the infection—like looking into the liver without a microscope. I always ask for a copy of my test results, and I keep my own file. It helps me feel as if I'm doing all I can on my end.

— Betsy

Enzymes. A liver cell produces enzymes that live within the cell or its membranes. In a way, you can think of your liver as a powerful chemical factory; it changes raw materials into the substances your body needs. Enzymes are catalysts that help a liver cell do its job of creating the specific chemical changes that give your body fuel to live. Here are the names of the enzymes you need to remember:

- **ALT (SGPT):** alanine aminotransferase
- **AST (SGOT):** aspartate aminotransferase
- **GGT:** gamma-glutamyl transferase
- **ALP:** alkaline phosphatase

By measuring the level of liver enzymes in your blood, doctors can monitor ongoing liver injury. How? Under normal conditions, the level of these enzymes in your bloodstream is relatively low. But when liver cells are injured, destroyed, or die, the liver cells becomes leaky, and the enzymes escape into the blood that is circulating through the liver. When liver cells are injured, liver enzyme levels in the blood rise. Therefore, the level of the enzymes in your blood correlates loosely with the severity of liver injury. Most patients with chronic hepatitis C have mild ongoing liver injury; in fact, ALT is normal in a high proportion of patients[36].

Patients tend to focus on their ALT and AST levels, but other tests, such as bilirubin, albumin, INR, platelet count, and MELD score, are more important in measuring the health and function of your liver.

Bilirubin. Bilirubin is a molecule that circulates in the blood, and is derived from the breakdown of the hemoglobin in red blood cells. It is normally taken up from the blood by a healthy liver. When the liver is diseased, bilirubin clearance decreases, and bilirubin levels in blood rise.

When the liver fails to take up and eliminate bilirubin from the blood, the skin and whites of the eyes turn yellow (jaundice), urine darkens, and the color of the bowel movement lightens (now you know why your doctor asks you probing questions about the color of your bowel movements). Jaundice usually implies severe liver injury or disease. Normal bilirubin is 1.2 milligrams or less per deciliter serum. Bilirubin is one of the tests used in the calculation of MELD score (see section in this chapter on MELD on page 33).

Albumin. Albumin is another protein that is synthesized (manufactured) by the liver. Liver cells secrete albumin to maintain the volume of blood in the arteries and veins. When albumin levels drop to extremely low levels, fluid may leak out of the blood vessels into the surrounding tissues. This causes swelling, known as edema. Normal albumin is 3.5 grams or more per deciliter serum. Edema tends to develop when levels drop below three grams per deciliter.

Unlike increases in liver enzyme, which occur within hours to days of the liver injury, albumin levels do not fall unless there has been chronic progressive liver injury for at least one month. This is because albumin has a long residence time in the plasma; its half-life is approximately 30 days. A decrease in serum albumin, therefore, reflects a slowly progressive, ongoing reduction in the liver's ability to synthesize this protein.

Be aware that there are also reasons unrelated to the liver that can cause a decrease in albumin, and your physician will take these into account when interpreting test results. Nonetheless, a significant, sustained decrease in serum albumin may indicate poor liver function and cirrhosis of the liver. Patients with very low albumin counts may need to be considered for liver transplantation.

Prothrombin Time (PT or INR). Remember our comparison of the liver to a chemical factory? The liver also synthesizes many proteins that maintain normal blood clotting. Prothrombin time (PT) or INR is the name of the most common test that measures a combination of blood clotting factors (proteins). If your INR increases, it means that your liver is not creating enough factors, so it takes your blood longer to clot. Normal INR is 1.0, and anything higher indicates that the liver is not creating enough prothrombin.

Unlike albumin, clotting factors can decrease rapidly—within days or even hours of a severe liver injury. In severe cases, clotting disturbances may signal the need for an early transplant. In patients with chronic hepatitis and chronic liver disease, a prolonged prothrombin time can be a warning that the liver is having trouble with its synthetic functions.

Typically, doctors will administer vitamin K, a vitamin essential for normal clotting factors, to determine whether the clotting disorder is reversible. Patients who have persistent, prolonged elevations in prothrombin time that do not respond to vitamin K have severe liver disease. INR is also one of the tests used in calculating your MELD score (see below).

Platelet Count. Platelet count is measured as part of a complete blood count. Platelets are blood elements that are important in maintaining normal clotting—low platelet count increases the risk of bleeding, especially during procedures. Patients with advanced liver disease or cirrhosis have an altered portal circulation (the conduit through which blood returns to the liver from the intestine and other abdominal organs) due to the scarring of the liver, which impedes flow through the portal vein and increases portal venous pressure. As a result, the spleen, which drains through the portal vein to the liver, becomes congested, and platelets are trapped in the spleen and removed from circulation. In addition, the liver synthesizes a hormone, thrombopoeitin, which stimulates the bone marrow to produce platelets. In patients with advanced liver disease, blood levels of thrombopoeitin fall, and the stimulus for production of platelets decreases. Because platelet count is related to both liver function and changes to the portal circulation, a drop in platelet count often signals a change in the course of liver disease and an increase in the risk for clinical complications. In fact, platelet count may be the single most useful blood test in early detection of cirrhosis.

MELD Score. MELD score may be the most important test for you to remember. MELD is used for patients with cirrhosis to predict 90-day survival, and is the basis for allocation of donor organs for liver transplantation[37, 38, 39, 40, 41, 42]. MELD is calculated from bilirubin, INR, and creatinine, and ranges from 6 to 40. If you know the results of your bilirubin, INR, and creatinine, you can calculate your MELD score (visit the website, www.mayoclinic.org/meld/mayomodel6.html, for more information). Patients with cirrhosis with MELD <10 typically are relatively stable, with little need for liver transplantation. Patients with MELD>40 die within 90 days, unless a transplant is performed. In most centers, patients are evaluated for liver transplantation when a MELD score ranges between 10 to 15 and are placed on the transplant waiting list when MELD is 15 or greater. In the United States, the average MELD at the time of transplantation is approximately 25.

Noninvasive Tests of Fibrosis. Fibrosis stage can also be estimated by biochemical blood tests and imaging methods, although the accuracy relative to liver biopsy is questionable[43]. The two imaging methods with the greatest promise to replace liver biopsy in assessment of fibrosis include transient elastography and magnetic resonance elastography. Nonetheless, the FDA has not yet approved elastography for liver fibrosis measurement[44].

Serum tests (such as FibroTest, FibroSure, HALT-C Model, and APRI) measuring a battery of blood components may also be useful in select patients. At least one serum test for fibrosis is currently FDA-approved, namely FibroTest. Serum tests are likely to be more accurate in assessing the extremes, ranging from patients with very severe fibrosis (cirrhosis) to those with very mild fibrosis (stage 0 to 1). Their performance, however, is not as good in distinguishing intermediate stages of fibrosis or for tracking changes over time[45].

Noninvasive Tests of Function. There are several methods for measuring various aspects of liver function. Tests relying on metabolism are reasonably accurate at the extremes of fibrosis[46], but they are less accurate in detecting intermediate stages of fibrosis[47].

Other tests that measure the portal circulation may be more informative. One of these tests involves administration of intravenous and oral cholates (a natural, endogenous compound called bile acid, which is synthesized in the liver from cholesterol[48]). In this test, the cholates are labeled with stable isotopes (not radioactive), and a 90-minute, timed blood sampling is conducted to test for cholate clearance. The tests quantify the percentage of the blood from the intestine and abdominal organs that is cleared by the liver. As liver disease worsens, clearance decreases, and shunt increases. These results correlate with the stage of fibrosis, and can identify patients at risk for clinical complications[49]. The FDA has not yet approved any of the noninvasive quantitative function tests.

Testing, Testing. In the past few years, I have seen the advancement in the specific new tests that help monitor your health. Yet all too often, I find that patients feel shut out by the complicated language of test results. Do not worry if you did not absorb every detail. Use these pages as a reference guide, and, for a more complete description of these tests, please refer to chapters 2 and 4 of the fifth edition of *Living with Hepatitis C: A Survivor's Guide.*

Always ask for copies of your tests. When you have questions, look up the explanations in these pages, and refer to the fifth edition of *Living with Hepatitis C: A Survivor's Guide.* Often, your physician can answer your questions and calm your fears if you voice them. Talk with your doctor.

Knowledge is power.

— Francis Bacon

3

PEGYLATED INTERFERON PLUS RIBAVIRIN

Backbone of Triple Therapy for HCV Genotype 1
Current Standard of Treatment for Non-1 HCV Genotypes

My first liver biopsy in 2006 showed cirrhosis, but I had no symptoms, and I was concerned about the side effects of interferon. Years later, I finally consulted a gastroenterologist about treatment. I asked him what my life expectancy would have been if I hadn't found out I had hepatitis C. He told me five years—if I was lucky. That brought me up short.

I was down. I thought I would die. I needed to do something, and treatment was my only choice. Luckily, I had infection with genotype 2—the easiest one to treat and cure. Within one month, while taking pegylated interferon and ribavirin, the HCV RNA was undetectable, and I stopped treatment after 6 months. Treatment was rough; I had a lot of side effects, but it was worth it. I'm now nine months after treatment, and the virus is still undetectable. My doctor is optimistic; he says I'm cured! My liver tests look good; nearly all of them continue to improve—my liver seems to be healing itself.

I'm glad I took the treatment. I've had hepatitis C since 1980—30 years—and this is the first time my liver has gotten a rest.

— Emma

EMMA WAS treated and cured of her hepatitis C through the combination of pegylated interferon plus ribavirin (PEGIFN/RBV). Many patients have been cured by this treatment, particularly the patients infected with HCV genotype 2. Even today, in 2011, the primary treatment for non-1 genotypes of HCV is PEGIFN/RBV[50].

Prior to May, 2011, the combination of PEGIFN/RBV was the standard of care for the treatment of all genotypes of HCV. In May 2011, triple therapy was approved by the FDA, and is now the standard of care for HCV genotype 1 infection[51]. Even so, the backbone of triple therapy is still PEGIFN/RBV.

PEGIFN/RBV remains the standard of care in the treatment of non-1 genotypes. If you are infected with non-1 HCV genotypes, you should consider treatment with this combination. In this chapter, I will explain, in detail, the treatment with the combination of PEGIFN/RBV.

Here are the topics that will be covered:
- Getting Yourself Ready for Treatment
    - Mood and Physical Activity
    - Remember: Alcohol and Hepatitis C Do Not Mix
    - Co-Existing Medical Conditions
    - Complementary and Alternative Medicines (CAM)
- Drugs, Treatment Regimens, and Outcomes
    - Drugs
    - Pegasys
    - PegIntron
    - Ribavirin
- Treatment Regimens and Outcomes
    - SVR = Cure! The Primary Goal of Treatment
    - PEGIFN/RBV: The Backbone of Triple Therapy for HCV Genotype 1
    - Pegasys Plus Ribavirin
    - PegIntron Plus Ribavirin
    - Dose of Ribavirin and Duration of Treatment
- Response-Guided Therapy
    - Rapid Virologic Response
    - The 12-Week Guideline
    - Factors Determining Response to PEGIFN/RBV

GETTING YOURSELF READY FOR TREATMENT

Mood and Physical Activity. As a patient with chronic hepatitis C, you may experience fatigue, loss of energy, loss of concentration, and a sense of inadequacy in performing your daily activities. These symptoms, feelings, and attitudes may make you emotional or susceptible to periods of depression. It is important for you to do all that you can to address these issues and correct problems prior to embarking on a course of therapy with PEGIFN/RBV. Some patients may require evaluation by a counselor, social worker, or psychiatrist, or initiation of antidepressant therapy for two to four weeks prior to starting antiviral treatment.

I encourage you to continue to remain physically active, pursue your occupation, socialize, and maintain proper nutrition. I also recommend regular exercise and a well-balanced diet supplemented with one multi-vitamin per day.

Remember: Alcohol and Hepatitis C Do Not Mix. Undoubtedly, you have been counseled to avoid excessive alcohol intake; the combination of alcohol and hepatitis C may accelerate your liver disease. In addition, your ability to respond to PEGIFN/RBV is impaired by the use of alcohol. Your chance for sustained virologic response decreases with increased alcohol use. For these reasons, I discourage the daily drinking of alcohol or consumption of large amounts at any time in all patients with chronic hepatitis C.

Co-Existing Medical Conditions. Pegylated interferon and ribavirin are potent medications that can stress your body. Severe anemia from ribavirin has been associated with angina (heart pain) and even heart attacks. If you are over 60 years of age, or have risk factors for coronary artery disease (such as smoking, high cholesterol, high blood pressure, diabetes mellitus, obesity, or positive family history), then cardiac stress testing is recommended prior to therapy. In rare cases, patients have experienced retinal hemorrhages on therapy, and risk factors for this complication include underlying diabetes mellitus or hypertension. An eye examination by an ophthalmologist may be warranted if you have diabetes or hypertension.

Complementary and Alternative Medicines (CAM). Patients commonly use over-the-counter products, supplements, herbal remedies, or alternative therapies[52]. A number of herbal remedies, teas, potions, over-the-counter products, and even acupuncture claim to be effective in treating liver disease and viral hepatitis, but none have been adequately studied or shown to be of proven benefit. I do not recommend CAM as an alternative to antiviral therapy to eradicate hepatitis C, because the effectiveness is doubtful, and the safety, in general, is unknown. Some have advocated use of CAM in patients taking PEGIFN/RBV in the hope that this approach will lessen side effects and improve adherence to the treatment regimen. Yet the effectiveness of CAM strategies in supporting patients through PEGIFN/RBV treatment remains unproven, and there is no evidence that CAM treatments improve your chances to achieve a cure of your hepatitis C. On the contrary, published reports implicate various CAM therapies in sporadic cases of severe liver injury. Be sure to check with your doctor before taking any over-the-counter products, herbal remedies, CAM therapies, or other substances.

DRUGS, TREATMENT REGIMENS, AND OUTCOMES

Two pegylated interferons, PegIntron and Pegasys with ribavirin, are FDA-approved for the treatment of chronic hepatitis C[53, 54, 55]. In the following discussion, I will focus on what you can expect in terms of virologic response and commonly encountered side effects from treatment with PEGIFN/RBV.

> *At first, I'd start to feel the side effects 24 to 48 hours after the injection. Now, three months later, the symptoms come on in 12 hours— instant flu.*
>
> *I think pegylated interferon has more residual effects than the doctors originally thought, because you're piling it up all the time.*
>
> — *Ray*

> *When I tried interferon monotherapy years ago, it felt as if I had the flu, but only for a week after the first injection. It wasn't so bad after that.*
>
> *Pegylated interferon is different. There's a slow buildup. It's cumulative, but I got better at compensating for the side effects.*
>
> — *Dan*

Drugs

Pegasys. The usual starting dose of Pegasys is 180 micrograms per week. The compound is pre-mixed, and is in solution in a preloaded syringe.

After Pegasys is injected, it slowly enters your bloodstream and takes 80 hours to reach peak concentrations in your blood. Your body slowly clears Pegasys; it takes 10 to 12 days to eliminate half of the drug. Most interferons are at least partially cleared from the body by passing through the kidneys into the urine. Pegasys, however, is too large to be filtered by the kidneys, and is not cleared by passage through the urine.

Instead, your body biodegrades the interferon, leaving the inert 40 kD PEG molecules to pass from the liver into bile and be eliminated from your system.

Blood concentrations remain fairly constant over the course of the week between injections. With multiple doses over the course of a year of treatment, Pegasys tends to accumulate in your body, and blood levels tend to increase[53, 55].

PegIntron. Dosage varies according to your weight: 1.5 micrograms of PegIntron per kilogram of body weight. For example, if you weigh 70 kilograms, you will inject 105 micrograms (70 kg x 1.5 micrograms/kg) of PegIntron weekly. PegIntron is also available in a prefilled syringe.

After PegIntron is injected, it takes 20 hours to reach peak concentrations in your blood. Your body eliminates half a dose of PegIntron in two to two-and-a-half days. In contrast to Pegasys, PegIntron is smaller, and approximately 30 percent is cleared through the kidneys. Like Pegasys, the interferon component of PegIntron is biodegraded by the body, and the 12 kD PEG is eliminated by passage from the liver into bile, and from the kidneys into urine.

There is a six-fold difference between the peak concentration and the lowest concentration achieved over the course of the week between injections. Compared to Pegasys, PegIntron has lower blood levels toward the end of the week prior to the next injection[54].

Despite the marked differences in pharmacokinetics of these two pegylated alfa interferons, the clinical responses are surprisingly very similar. Rates of sustained virologic response (SVR) are very similar for PegIntron compared to Pegasys when used as PEGIFN/RBV across HCV genotypes, HCV RNA levels, and stages of fibrosis.

Ribavirin. There are three formulations of ribavirin for oral dosing: Copegus (used with Pegasys), Rebetol (used with PegIntron), and Ribapak. Copegus and Rebetol are formulated as 200 milligram tablets. Ribapak is formulated in 400 and 600 milligram doses, and is distributed in a blisterpak.

The prescribed dosage of ribavirin varies by HCV genotype and weight. For HCV genotype 1 (and HCV genotypes 4, 5, 6), the dosage is 1,000 milligrams per day for a body weight of 75 kilograms or less, or 1,200 milligrams per day for a body weight of more than 75 kilograms. For HCV genotypes 2 and 3, less ribavirin is needed (only 800 milligrams per day). Nonetheless, higher ribavirin dosage—1,000 to 1,200 milligrams per day—may be advisable for HCV genotypes 2 and 3, if the planned treatment course is less than 24 weeks.

The dosages for Pegasys, PegIntron, and ribavirin that are described above are also the dosages used as the backbone for triple therapy with telaprevir or boceprevir (see chapters 4 and 5).

Treatment Regimens and Outcomes

SVR = Cure! The Primary Goal of Treatment. The primary goal of HCV treatment is to achieve sustained virologic response (SVR), which is defined as undetectable HCV RNA at 12 weeks (current sensitive assays for HCV RNA), or 24 weeks (past, less sensitive assays for HCV RNA) after the end of treatment. Studies of patients who achieved SVR, regardless of the type of treatment, indicate less than a 1 percent chance for relapse of HCV infection in over 10 years of follow-up. Patients achieving SVR are *cured* of their HCV infection, and are less likely to suffer complications of liver disease[56].

PEGIFN/RBV: The Backbone of Triple Therapy for HCV Genotype 1. PEGIFN/RBV is no longer the standard of care for HCV genotype 1. Triple therapy, using PEGIFN/RBV with either telaprevir or boceprevir, is the current standard for this HCV genotype. Because PEGIFN/RBV is considered a backbone of triple therapy, you need to become familiar with the outcomes and side effects of this combination, even if you are infected with HCV genotype 1.

Data from three large clinical trials of the combination of peginterferon with ribavirin are highlighted in Figures 3A and 3B.

FIGURE 3A: RATES OF SVR WITH PEGINTERFERON/RIBAVIRIN IN TREATMENT-NAÏVE PATIENTS

HCV GENOTYPE I   HCV GENOTYPES 2 AND 3

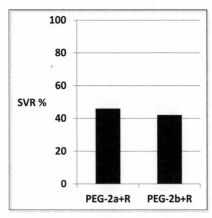
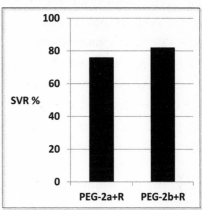

FIGURE 3A: The published rates of sustained virologic response (SVR) using peginterferon/ribavirin therapy are approximately 40 percent for HCV genotype 1 (left panel), and 80 percent for genotypes 2/3 (right panel)[53, 54]. PEG-2a is PEGASYS, and PEG-2b is PEGINTRON; R is ribavirin.

Pegasys Plus Ribavirin. In the FDA registration trial for Pegasys/Ribavirin[53], HCV genotypes were the major determinants for rates of sustained virologic response (SVR) to Pegasys plus ribavirin (Figure 3A). Patients with HCV genotype 1 had an SVR of 46 percent, and patients with HCV genotypes 2 and 3 had an SVR of 76 percent.

Side Effects. Common symptoms included fatigue, headache, sleeplessness, nausea, arthralgia (joint pains), fever, muscle aches, and rigors (shaking, chills). One in five patients also experienced depression.

PegIntron Plus Ribavirin. In the FDA registration trial for PegIntron/Ribavirin[54], HCV genotypes were, once again, the major determinants for rates of sustained virologic response to PegIntron plus ribavirin (Figure 3A). Patients with HCV genotype 1 had sustained responses of 42 percent, and patients with HCV genotypes 2 and 3 had sustained responses of 82 percent.

Side Effects. Side effects of PegIntron plus ribavirin were similar to those observed with Pegasys plus ribavirin. The most common side effects were flu-like symptoms, mood alteration, depression, fever, nausea, and injection-site reactions. Results with PegIntron and Pegasys are very similar; the table below depicts the range of results seen across PegIntron and Pegasys studies.

Genotypes	Likelihood of SVR during PEGIFN/RBV
1	42 to 46%
2 & 3	76 to 82%

Note: The table above reflects the combined likelihood of SVR for both Pegasys and PegIntron.

Dose of Ribavirin and Duration of Treatment. One trial of Pegasys[55] examined the dose of ribavirin and duration of treatment required for optimum treatment of HCV genotypes (Figure 3B). The findings of this trial remain the basis for current use of peginterferon/ribavirin:

- Genotype 1 requires high doses of ribavirin (1.0 to 1.2 grams per day, or g/d)
- Genotype 1 requires long duration of treatment (48 weeks)
- Genotypes 2 and 3 can be treated at lower doses of ribavirin (0.8 g/d)
- Genotypes 2 and 3 can be treated for shorter duration (24 weeks)

FIGURE 3B: EFFECT OF TREATMENT DURATION AND
RIBAVIRIN DOSE IN TREATMENT–NAÏVE PATIENTS

HCV GENOTYPE I   HCV GENOTYPES 2 AND 3

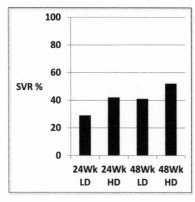
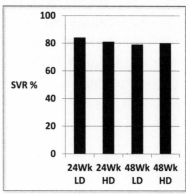

FIGURE 3B: Optimal results for HCV genotype 1 (left panel) require longer duration of treatment (48 weeks—48 Wk) and higher doses (HD) of ribavirin. A shorter
course (24 Wk) and lower dose (LD) ribavirin is sufficient for HCV genotypes 2
and 3 (right panel)[55].

Side Effects. There are two main side effects of ribavirin: decrease of red
blood cells (anemia) due to hemolysis (red cell breakdown), and rash.
Generally, these side effects are managed by reducing the dose of ribavirin,
but, occasionally, the anemia may require treatment with erythropoietin
analogue (EPO) or transfusion of blood.

RESPONSE-GUIDED THERAPY

On-treatment virologic response is a major predictor of SVR in patients
treated with PEGIFN/RBV[50]. Patients who clear rapidly have the
greatest chance for SVR. The definitions described below apply only to
PEGIFN/RBV treatment, and may not be appropriate when discussing
virologic responses during telaprevir-based or boceprevir-based triple
therapy. Separate definitions of virologic response and stop guidelines
have been developed for triple therapy, and are discussed in chapter 5.

Rapid Virologic Response. Rapid virologic response (RVR) is defined as undetectable HCV RNA at week four of PEGIFN/RBV. Patients who achieve RVR on PEGIFN/RBV have an 88 to 100 percent chance to achieve SVR, and may be candidates for a shorter duration of treatment. Patients with genotype 1 infection who experience rapid virologic response may require only 24 weeks of treatment, and those infected with HCV genotypes 2 or 3 who experience RVR may require as little as 12 weeks. On the other hand, the likelihood of RVR is much lower for HCV genotype 1 compared to other HCV genotypes:

Genotypes	Likelihood of RVR during PEGIFN/RBV
1	16%
2	71%
3	60%

The 12-Week Guideline. The level of HCV RNA at week 12 of PEGIFN/RBV defines the on-treatment response:

- Complete Early Virologic Response (cEVR): Undetectable HCV RNA
- Partial Early Virologic Response (pEVR): more than a 100-fold ($2\log_{10}$) drop from baseline, but still detectable HCV RNA
- Null Response: Less than 100-fold ($2\log_{10}$) drop in HCV RNA from baseline

Patients with cEVR have the highest likelihood of achieving SVR. In contrast, patients with null response are not likely to achieve SVR. Treatment is stopped in patients with null response (this is known as the 12-week stopping rule).

The Null Response. I will illustrate the null response further with the following example. If your baseline HCV RNA level was 2,000,000 copies per milliliter prior to treatment, the HCV RNA level must drop below 20,000 copies per milliliter of blood by week 12 in order for you to have a reasonable chance to clear HCV. If, by week 12, your HCV RNA has not fallen 100-fold, and remains above 20,000 copies per milliliter of blood, your chance for sustained virologic response (even if you continue treatment for a full 48 weeks) is less than 2 percent. In this case, the standard recommendation would be to discontinue treatment at week 12.

Factors Determining Response to PEGIFN/RBV. Rapid virologic response during PEGIFN/RBV is the single strongest predictor of achieving SVR. Several pre-treatment characteristics or factors may impair response to PEGIFN/RBV[57]. These include:

- Obesity and insulin resistance
- Hepatic steatosis (fatty liver)
- Advanced fibrosis or cirrhosis
- African American race
- Latino ethnicity
- Non-1 HCV genotypes
- High levels of HCV RNA
- Active substance abuse (alcohol, drugs)

A genetic test that measures your ability to respond to interferon is the polymorphism of the IL28B gene[58]. This test yields results of your genes, and the results are given as CC, CT, or TT, which are linked to the ability to respond to interferon. IL28B polymorphism is the major pre-treatment predictor of response to PEGIFN/RBV, and accounts for most of the differences in SVR between races and ethnicities. Patients with HCV genotype 1 and the IL28B genotype CC have a 60 to 80 percent chance for SVR when treated with PEGIFN/RBV, while patients with CT or TT genotypes have only a 20 to 30 percent chance for SVR.

THE PATIENTS' EXPERIENCES

With my first dose, I had the worst side effects ever. My teeth were chattering, and I had a fever. But by the next week, it wasn't as bad.

— Ed

Although I had a lot of the same side effects I had when I took Rebetron, everything started improving after I learned I was virus-free. My hair doesn't come out in handfuls anymore. Body aches are down, and the fatigue is a little better.

— Delores

The first dose was not as bad as regular interferon. I compare myself to others who are really sick, or so tired they can't do anything. It didn't make me feel like that.

— Ben

I take my shot on Monday night. On Tuesday or Wednesday, I get the reaction: a temperature, achy muscles. I take Tylenol®, and, by the next morning, I'm fine.

— Rhonda

When I took the first dose, I got chills and nausea. I went into work, and I started shaking. My teeth were chattering. I had the sweats. I missed three days of work, so I called the nurse and said I can't handle this. I can't miss work.

The nurse was a big help. She encouraged me. After the second shot, my body got used to it. But I didn't like having dry, itchy skin, especially around the injection areas, and the tiredness and depression. I felt like a martyr.

Why did I stick with it? I try to keep my word. If I tell someone I'm going to do something, I do it—and a year later, my blood tests show that the virus is still undetectable.

— Tom

I'd get tired if I carried groceries from the car to the house. The doctor thought that maybe I'd have to cut back on work, but I never did. Treatment did not interfere with my work, daily functions, or my family, at all.

— Alice

It's unbelievable to deal with your emotions. Every week they mutate, like the virus. Every week is different.

— David

I have a blue-collar mentality. My dad always said a little hard work never killed anybody. So, when I can't go out and do stuff, I feel bad.

The sprinkler broke. I got all my tools out. Where do you think they all are two months later? Still in the same place. I had to fix the pump or the lawn would die, but I had no energy, no will to put the tools back. It's a mental thing.

— Shawn

I call it "the day-after-the-shot day." It's pretty dramatic. That's when I have most of my body aches and pains. I can't function. I go to bed after work at five o'clock. I'm doing better now; I can stay up until eight o'clock.

— Michelle

I started at a high dose, but it was reduced because of my blood counts. The treatment wasn't agreeing with me, but I had no side effects: no fatigue, no weight loss. The only thing I can recall was the itching that started around six months. No rash, but I'd itch like crazy on the lower part of my ankles, legs, and the back of my neck.

— Paul

The hardest part was trying to communicate what treatment is like to my family and friends. I had a hard time with that; with getting them to understand that I can't go out, that I'm exhausted, and it wouldn't be any fun.

I've had hepatitis C for 30 years, and I think their attitude is, "What's new? Why are you whining?"

— Jody

I responded. That was the wonderful part. I didn't expect it after other courses of therapy and a diagnosis of cirrhosis. Then I got a rash so bad, I had to quit taking ribavirin. It was all over my body—even in my mouth—and so painful, I couldn't sleep.

I thought that without ribavirin, pegylated interferon alone wouldn't clear the virus, but it did.

— Ted

I'd have a red spot where I injected the needle for a few days after the injection. Then it would go away. Over the year, the red spots turned black. I'd have black marks on my thighs. I refused to wear shorts. Two to three months after, I was done with treatment; they totally went away.

— Clara

I didn't go to church for six months. I just slept. It's a miracle I didn't lose my business. God had His hand in it.

— Dottie

Pegylated? It was Greek to me when I started. You get an education as you go. I was very optimistic; glad to have hope.

— Sam

I felt blessed. That's as good a word as any. I never felt I was particularly deserving of anything special. Why was I picked to be someone who responded?

I'm the head of a national sales force. A lot of people were depending on me to keep them from being laid off when the company went through a period of turmoil while I was on treatment. I felt like a shepherd with a flock. I couldn't let them down. Maybe that's why I got the extra strength.

— Mike

I didn't clear the virus, but a recent biopsy showed that the inflammation and fibrosis improved. My liver went from stage II back to stage I.

— Josh

Myalgia kept me awake. I had this gnawing, irritating grinding in my muscles. The doctor put me on sleep medicine. I was so desperate for sleep.

It worked, and with no hangover, too. It just shut my mind off, so I only took it at home. I had no problem getting off it after treatment.

— Mandy

I said, "Well, okay, I did not respond to the medicine. But it's not over yet, because the Great Physician, God, is still at work, and I am not giving up." I refuse to believe that I will have to live the rest of my life with this virus inside me.

— Ken

I didn't think regular interferon was a big deal. I wouldn't say that about pegylated interferon and ribavirin, but I've never gotten to the point where I can't function.

— Mary

I filled out this form that asked me if I felt good or bad. I don't feel either. My sexual desire is gone. I feel like a machine. I do things because I have to do them.

— *Mel*

The first test showed I was responding. Anybody who is going to take this treatment has to be committed. I've thought about quitting, but giving up would be worse. I've had hepatitis C since 1988, and I want to get rid of it.

— *Jay*

Treatment made me more compassionate. I used to avoid people who were suffering from other diseases, because I didn't know what to say. Now, I go right up to them, and I ask them how they're really doing.

— *Carol*

I call it my bath therapy: soaking in a tub with mineral salts. It really helps me relax.

— *Cammy*

I try not to think about the side effects. I look at the end result and keep my eyes on the prize.

I had to rearrange my thinking around an emotional, mental wall. I hadn't talked to anyone until I confided in a friend who had cancer and chemotherapy. I'm lucky I picked him, because he knows exactly what I'm going through.

Once I found out I was in remission, there was hope. So I finally told my dad.

— *Terry*

If I walk up a flight of stairs, I'm huffing and puffing, because ribavirin lowers your oxygen. I have to stop on the landing and take deep breaths to get more air into my system.

— Kendra

I try very hard to take a nap in my car at lunchtime. It helps me get through the workday.

— Sara

I work full time. I was raised to think that, when you quit, that's when you die. So you just keep going. When both my white and red blood counts dropped, I was doing what I had to do, but I was in a total fog. My boss said, "You're going to have to start writing things down."

The doctors reduced my doses of both interferon and ribavirin, and I went on an antidepressant. That helped.

— Mindy

I took baths in an Aveeno® bath treatment with oatmeal powder for the itching, and I used their anti-itch cream, too.

— Marcia

Baking soda and water worked as well as anything for the itching.

— Jill

I'm exhausted all the time. I go to bed at seven o'clock at night, and get up at seven o'clock in the morning. I'm rarely up to see the sunset.

Exercise helps. At first, I got tired, but, now, I'm doing better. I started with nine holes of golf, and I've worked my way up to 18.

— George

I run out of gas, and I feel spaced out. I enjoy a nap now and then.

— Rosa

I never missed a day of work. I took the meds with me when I had to travel, icing them down.

I'd also time my shots. I started on Friday, and I'd have 36 hours with aches, pains, and headaches. By the time Monday came, I was feeling alright to work. I could do routine stuff. By Wednesday, I was feeling like myself again. I would plan complicated projects on Thursday and Friday when I was mentally sharper.

— Marcus

I was always cold. It felt like I stayed cold for the whole 48 weeks of treatment. I never put on shorts that year. Instead, I wore insulated jeans.

— Jose

I drink a lot of water. I have water bottles everywhere: at home, at work. I never drink pop. I only drink filtered water.

— Tina

I don't concentrate as well on this interferon, so I use a hand-held computer. I set it to buzz me when it's time to take the ribavirin. Then, on the screen, it asks me if I took it, and I have to insert "yes." I've never missed any ribavirin or injections.

— Manuel

I'd get redness at the site of the injection, but I learned to rotate the injection sites; move the needle around. The redness went away after a couple of months.

— Bill

*My faith and spirituality help me through it. I have wonderful church
support with people praying for my healing.*

— Marcia

*"One day at a time." I never understood that saying until the doctor
told me I only had five years left. "Okay," I thought, "I'd better take that
cruise now." When I think of something I always wanted to do, and I
can afford it, I do it now. I even went parasailing last May!*

— Ty

*I look at it this way: the rash is ugly, but the fact that I have it means
that at least my body knows something is going on.*

— Sandra

*I'm very conscious of what I eat. I cut back on sweets, junk food, and I
eat a lot of fruit with fiber. I also drink lots of water and apple, cranberry,
and orange juice. I even juice my own apples and veggies.*

—Jane

SPECIAL CONSIDERATIONS

African Americans. ViraHepC was the first clinical trial of PEGIFN/
RBV that was specifically designed to assess the effectiveness of this
treatment in African Americans[59]. In this study, all patients were infected
with HCV genotype 1, and an equal number of African Americans and
Caucasian patients with chronic hepatitis C were compared. Sustained
virologic responses were 28 percent in African Americans versus 50 percent in Caucasians (Figure 3C). Doses and duration of medications were
similar between African Americans and Caucasian patients.

One reason for the lower rate of SVR is African Americans have a
much lower prevalence of the IL28B genotype CC, and a higher prevalence of the IL28B genotype TT. The CC genotype is associated with a

greater likelihood of spontaneous clearance of HCV after acute infection, and a greater likelihood of SVR in response to interferon. IL28B polymorphisms are discussed in greater detail in the chapters on triple therapy (chapters 4 and 5) and future treatments (chapter 6).

FIGURE 3C: VIROLOGIC RESPONSES IN AFRICAN AMERICANS VS WHITES: TREATMENT-NAÏVE PATIENTS

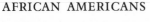

AFRICAN AMERICANS   WHITES

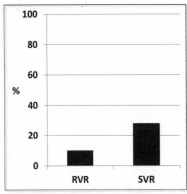
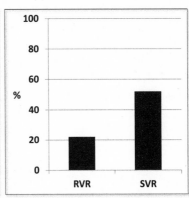

FIGURE 3C: The virologic responses to peginterferon/ribavirin of African Americans and white Americans infected with HCV genotype 1 are compared[59]. On-treatment (RVR, rapid virologic response) and sustained virologic (SVR) responses are lower in African Americans.

Cirrhosis. Patients with cirrhosis in clinical trials typically have a clinically stable disease, lack history of varices (large veins in the esophagus or other parts of the GI (gastrointestinal) tract due to liver disease), ascites, or encephalopathy, and have a nearly normal laboratory profile. Study patients with cirrhosis are "compensated," which means they lack clinical or lab evidence of advanced liver disease. Rates of SVR are consistently lower in patients with cirrhosis, regardless of the antiviral treatment. The lower rate of SVR in patients with cirrhosis compared to patients without cirrhosis has been observed in trials of interferon, pegylated interferon, PEGIFN/RBV, and, now, even triple therapy.

We treated sicker patients who had experienced complications of liver disease, many of whom were ultimately listed and underwent transplantation. These patients had early decompensation (experienced clinical or laboratory evidence of severe liver disease). The regimen that we used, LADR (Low Accelerating Dose Regimen), started at low doses, and gradually increased both interferon and ribavirin. Only 24 percent of all these patients, and 13 percent of patients infected with HCV genotype 1, achieved sustained virologic response[60].

In the HALT-C trial of re-treatment of nonresponders to prior interferon or interferon plus ribavirin with PEGIFN/RBV, sustained virologic response in those with fibrosis and the least severe disease was 23 percent, but only 9 percent in those with cirrhosis and the most severe disease[61].

In LADR-A2ALL (Adult-to-Adult Liver Donor Liver Transplant Study presented at AASLD 2009), a similar poor response to PEGIFN/ RBV was observed: SVR of 22 percent in HCV genotype 1 and 31 percent in HCV genotype 2/3. Trials in this patient population, using new direct-acting antiviral therapy, are planned.

Treatment of patients with cirrhosis requires close supervision and frequent monitoring of laboratory tests. Complications, such as infection, bleeding, worsening ascites, and encephalopathy, may arise either due to an underlying severity of disease or the effects of treatment[62, 63, 64]. In such cases, early intervention is warranted. For these reasons, treating patients with cirrhosis who have had clinical decompensation should only be done in liver centers or by physicians with extensive experience in the treatment of patients with chronic hepatitis C and the management of advanced liver disease. Some considerations prior to treating patients with cirrhosis include evaluation and eradication of varices by endo-scopic ligation therapy, prophylactic antibiotics to prevent spontaneous bacterial peritonitis, and the use of pre-emptive lactulose, neomycin, or rifaximine to reduce risk of encephalopathy.

Renal Failure. Patients with renal failure, especially those on dialysis, have an increased prevalence of infection with chronic hepatitis C. Generally, patients with renal failure respond well to interferon, and have a sustained virologic response to interferon or pegylated interferon monotherapy that is equivalent (or even superior) to patients with chronic hepatitis C without renal failure. Kidney dysfunction, however, does impair the excretion of ribavirin, leading to its accumulation in blood and tissue, which, in turn, leads to anemia (hemolysis), bone marrow suppression, and mucosal and skin injury. Current studies suggest that rates of SVR in patients with renal failure (even those on dialysis) may be improved by the addition of low doses of ribavirin (200 to 400 milligrams every other day). If ribavirin is used, it is typically administered at very low doses under careful supervision by an experienced physician.

AFTER TREATMENT: WHAT NEXT?

If You Achieved SVR. A sustained virologic response (SVR) is the most desirable outcome after antiviral treatment, and indicates that you likely have been *cured* of HCV infection. Patients with SVR have cleared the virus from their blood, and most have improvement in their liver biopsy (fewer inflammatory cells and less damage). Long-term follow-up of sustained responders (for more than 10 years) indicates that relapse rarely, if ever, occurs: less than 1 percent chance of late relapse. Once you have achieved SVR, you are very likely cured of hepatitis C, and are at a lower risk for future complications[65, 66].

If you had advanced fibrosis or cirrhosis prior to treatment, you may still be at risk for liver cancer even after you have achieved SVR[56]. I recommend continued surveillance for liver cancer through your physician. Surveillance strategies vary, but a common strategy incorporates ultrasonography of the liver every 6 to 12 months.

If You Relapsed or Had Nonresponse to PEGIFN/RBV. If you still harbor HCV infection, you are at risk for disease progression, the development of cirrhosis and its complications, and liver cancer. If you are infected with HCV genotype 1, you should consider evaluation for re-treatment with triple therapy (see chapters 4 and 5). If you are infected with non-1 HCV genotypes, your options for re-treatment may be limited to participation in clinical trials. Telaprevir and boceprevir may have activity against HCV genotype 2, but seem to have little, if any, activity against HCV genotype 3 (see chapter 5 concerning re-treatment of non-1 HCV genotypes with triple therapy).

The greatest need for re-treatment is in patients with more advanced fibrosis or cirrhosis upon liver biopsy, because they have the greatest risk for future clinical complications. Nonetheless, the decision to offer re-treatment is based upon the vigor of your prior response to PEGIFN/RBV and other factors (see chapter 5).

Whether you decide on re-treatment with triple therapy or not, routine blood testing and clinical follow-up through your physician and healthcare providers are advisable.

GENERAL CONSIDERATIONS

Alcohol. You should understand that the continued use of alcohol can cause early progression to cirrhosis and liver failure. Also, in planning for the future and need for potential treatments, you should be aware that ongoing alcohol use is a contraindication to liver transplantation. If you need a liver transplant, but are drinking alcohol, you will not be approved for the transplant. A person infected with HCV should abstain from alcohol use.

Smoking. Smoking is not only deleterious to your overall health, but it may also increase your risk of liver cancer. Smoking may also be a contraindication to liver transplantation. Avoid cigarettes.

Vaccinations. The National Institutes of Health (NIH) guidelines indicate that hepatitis C patients should undergo vaccination against both hepatitis A and B. Both vaccines are safe and highly effective in preventing infection, and the two vaccines may now be co-administered (TWINRIX®). Check with your physician about vaccination.

CONCLUDING REMARKS

PEGIFN/RBV was the standard of care in the treatment of all patients with chronic hepatitis C up to May, 2011. Then triple therapy became the new standard, but only for HCV genotype 1. Patients infected with non-1 HCV genotypes represent about 25 percent of cases of chronic hepatitis C, and PEGIFN/RBV is still the current recommended treatment for this subgroup of patients. High rates of SVR of approximately 80 percent are achievable in HCV genotypes 2 and 3 with PEGIFN/ RBV, but without any of the new antiviral drugs for HCV. It is important to remember the effectiveness and utility of the old standards as the treatment paradigm shifts toward new therapeutic options.

No physician, insofar as he is a physician, considers his own good in what he prescribes, but the good of his patient.

— *Plato*

4

CANDIDATES FOR TRIPLE THERAPY

What Is Triple Therapy?
Should I Be Treated with Triple Therapy?

I believe alternative therapies might be helpful, but they won't cure this very potent virus that is constantly mutating in your body. I advise a strong pharmaceutical approach. Drugs like telaprevir and boceprevir have more than a 70 percent cure rate, and are the best we have at the moment. I have the type 1A hepatitis C, and it seems to be the hardest to cure. My advice to anyone considering the treatment is to try it now. Those two drugs became FDA approved in 2011. Hopefully, if treated, you'll be in the 70 percent or more who will be cured. Before I sought treatment, I didn't have any knowledge of what was out there. My doctor felt very positive about the new antivirals that work directly on the virus and in the liver. He felt I was well-suited for the new class of antivirals.

— Frank

A NEW era of therapy for HCV genotype 1 has arrived. As of May, 2011, the new standard of care is now triple therapy, the combination of boceprevir or telaprevir with peginterferon/ribavirin[67, 68, 69, 70, 71]. For patients infected with HCV genotype 1, triple therapy promises to increase the chance to clear HCV infection.

Approximately 20 years ago, the agent of nonA–nonB hepatitis, hepatitis C, was discovered, and the first treatment, non-pegylated interferon monotherapy, was approved by the FDA[72, 73, 74, 75]. Since then, rates of sustained virologic response (SVR) in patients with HCV genotype 1 infection steadily improved: from approximately 5 percent with interferon monotherapy[75] to 45 percent with peginterferon/ribavirin[53, 54, 55]. Triple therapy ushers in the next leap forward in antiviral therapy, as rates of SVR for patients with HCV genotype 1 infection should now approach 75 percent.

In this chapter, I introduce you to the drugs that comprise triple therapy. I also discuss the various factors to consider when making a decision to proceed with treatment. I provide guidelines for the use of FDA-approved triple therapies based on the first generation inhibitors of the HCV NS3/4A protease, boceprevir and telaprevir. Direct-acting antivirals against HCV have arrived. The future is now.

In this chapter I will answer the following questions:

- Why Should I Be Treated?
    - You may have significant liver disease even if you have no symptoms.
    - Hepatitis C *can* be cured.
- What Is Triple Therapy?
    - Triple therapy includes three drugs: peginterferon, ribavirin, and either boceprevir or telaprevir.
    - Peginterferon is injected beneath the skin.
    - Ribavirin is taken by mouth.
    - Boceprevir and telaprevir are also taken by mouth. They are the first FDA-approved medicines that directly block the HCV life cycle.

- I've Heard That Interferon Has a Lot of Side Effects. Why Not Treat Me with Just Boceprevir or Telaprevir?
  - You cannot clear HCV from your body if you take boceprevir or telaprevir alone.
  - You may develop resistant HCV if you take boceprevir or telaprevir alone.
- Am I a Candidate for Triple Therapy?
  - See your doctor and get evaluated.
  - Contraindications
  - Triple therapy is primarily for HCV genotype 1 infection.
  - Triple therapy is more effective than peginterferon/ribavirin in the treatment of African Americans.
  - Triple therapy is more effective than peginterferon/ribavirin in the treatment of patients with fibrosis or cirrhosis.
- My Doctor Told Me That the Use of Triple Therapy in My Case Would Be Off Label. What Is Off Label?
  - Use of triple therapy if you are a person with:
    - Non-1 HCV genotypes
    - Decompensated cirrhosis
    - Liver transplantation
    - Co-infection with HIV and HCV
    - A child with chronic HCV infection
- Can You Test My Blood Before Treatment to See If I Will Respond to Triple Therapy?
- Concluding Remarks

WHY SHOULD I BE TREATED?

This is a common question. You may have had chronic hepatitis C for many years, but you lack symptoms, feel healthy, have normal laboratory values, and lead an active, productive life. You just do not feel a pressing need for therapy, especially a therapy with significant side effects. In addition, you may have heard through the grapevine that hepatitis C cannot be cured. Let me attempt to dispel these myths.

You May Have Significant Liver Disease Even If You Have No Symptoms. One myth concerning hepatitis C is the disease is mild and will not alter a person's life—after all, hepatitis C was originally called nonA, nonB hepatitis: in other words, a non-disease. We now know that hepatitis C is potentially very serious, and may lead to liver failure, liver cancer, and death from liver disease.[76] Hepatitis C is the leading indicator for liver transplantation in the United States. A major reason to consider therapy is the fact that hepatitis C can be a chronically progressive disease that can shorten your life or cause you significant harm, resulting in the need for medical treatments or even liver transplantation. You may be at risk even if you lack symptoms, and have a normal physical examination and laboratory tests[36].

Hepatitis C *Can* Be Cured. Another common myth that will influence your decision to be treated may be your perception that hepatitis C cannot be cured. On the contrary, hepatitis C *can* be cured. The primary goal of your treatment is to achieve sustained virologic response (SVR), which is defined as undetectable HCV RNA in your blood 12 to 24 weeks after the end of therapy. If you achieve SVR, you have greater than 99 percent likelihood (99 chances out of 100) for long-term clearance of HCV RNA for over 10 years, in which case I would suggest to you that you are likely cured of HCV[77] (Figure 4A). In fact, most hepatologists now accept SVR as essentially virologic cure. SVR means that the HCV has disappeared, and is not likely to ever re-emerge.

Clearing HCV (SVR) has major benefits. SVR reduces fibrosis (scarring) in your liver and lowers your risk to clinically deteriorate, develop cirrhosis and its complications, and die from liver failure or require liver transplantation[56, 65, 66]. You should consider therapy for chronic hepatitis C because you can clear the infection and halt or even reverse your liver disease.

FIGURE 4A: ACHIEVING SVR EQUALS CURE IN NEARLY ALL CASES

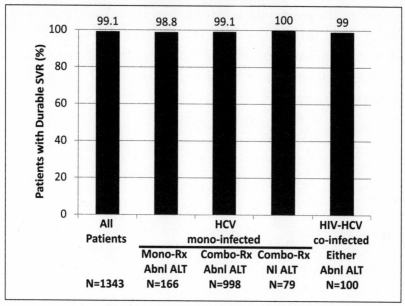

Swain MG, et al. Gastroenterology 2010;139:1593-1601.

FIGURE 4A: Patients achieving SVR, regardless of treatment regimen or HIV co-infection, remain free of hepatitis C in follow-up for up to 10 years[77].

WHAT IS TRIPLE THERAPY?

Triple Therapy Includes Three Drugs: Peginterferon, Ribavirin, and Either Boceprevir or Telaprevir. The drugs used in triple therapy of HCV include the combination of peginterferon and ribavirin with either boceprevir (VICTRELIS®) or telaprevir (INCIVEK®). You may be wondering, "How difficult is the treatment?" The treatment is:

- Peginterferon injection weekly,
- Ribavirin, two to three pills twice daily, plus
- Boceprevir (four pills) or telaprevir (two pills) three times a day

You have to take a shot once a week and several pills each day for 24 to 48 weeks. To aid absorption from the intestine, you must have a meal with each dose of boceprevir and telaprevir. It is very important that you take your medicines as prescribed, on schedule, and without missing doses. Why? If you miss doses, the treatment is less likely to clear HCV, and you would be more likely to develop resistant forms of HCV. If you develop resistant HCV, you may not be able to be treated in the future with other drugs similar to boceprevir and telaprevir that inhibit the HCV NS3/4A protease.

Peginterferon Is Injected Beneath the Skin. You will be taught to self-administer weekly subcutaneous injections of peginterferon (under the skin using a syringe with a very small needle). The dose of peginterferon will vary according to the type of peginterferon and your body weight. There are two formulations of peginterferon, Pegasys and PegIntron. Pegasys is administered at a fixed dose (180 micrograms per week), and PegIntron dosage is based on your body weight (1.5 micrograms/kilogram per week).

Ribavirin Is Taken By Mouth. Ribavirin pills are taken twice a day, and doses and the number of pills vary with HCV genotype and body weight. There are three main formulations of ribavirin for treating HCV, Rebetol, Copegus, and Ribapak. For Rebetol and Copegus, the pill size is 200 milligrams, and the usual ribavirin prescription is 600 milligrams or three pills twice daily. Pill burden can be reduced by use of pill sizes from 400 to 600 milligrams (as is the case with Ribapak).

Boceprevir and Telaprevir Are Also Taken By Mouth. They Are the First FDA-Approved Medicines That Directly Block the HCV Life Cycle. Boceprevir (200 milligrams per pill) is prescribed as 800 milligrams or four pills every eight hours. In various treatment regimens, the duration of boceprevir may vary from 24 to 44 weeks. Telaprevir (375 milligrams per pill) is prescribed as 750 milligrams or two pills every eight hours. The duration of telaprevir is always 12 weeks. Whether you are prescribed boceprevir or telaprevir, you will take the peginterferon injections weekly, and ribavirin pills twice daily for 24 to 48 weeks. You must eat a meal with each dose of either bocepre-vir or telaprevir. With telaprevir, a fatty meal of at least 300 calories is required.

I had some nausea, but only vomited once. The protocol required eating 300 calories every eight hours. That meant I had to get out of bed to eat, and take my telaprevir at the right time—being awakened by my alarm in the middle of sleep was aggravating. One time, my beeper went off to remind me to eat while I was interviewing a potential employee about a job. Poor guy, he thought the beeper indicated the end of the interview, so he stopped talking, and left the interview early. Fortunately, he was a great recruit, and got the job anyway.

— *Barb*

I'VE HEARD THAT INTERFERON HAS A LOT OF SIDE EFFECTS. WHY NOT TREAT ME WITH JUST BOCEPREVIR OR TELAPREVIR?

You Cannot Clear HCV From Your Body If You Take Boceprevir or Telaprevir Alone. All three drugs within the triple therapy com-bination are important, and are required for maximal effectiveness. You should view triple therapy as one treatment, where the three drugs work together to give you the best chance to clear HCV[78].

Monotherapy (treatment with boceprevir or telaprevir alone) is not advised. If you take boceprevir or telaprevir alone, the HCV RNA in your blood will decrease over the first few days, but remain detect-able, and, later, begin to increase within 14 days.[79] This rebound or rise in HCV RNA represents the emergence of HCV that is resistant to boceprevir and telaprevir, making SVR impossible to achieve. You have essentially zero chance to clear HCV and nearly 100 percent chance to develop resistant HCV if you take boceprevir or telaprevir alone.

WARNING: Never treat with boceprevir or telaprevir alone. When using these drugs to treat HCV, they must always be taken in a regimen that includes peginterferon and ribavirin.

You May Develop Resistant HCV If You Take Boceprevir or Telaprevir Alone. In the preceding section, I told you that the emergence of HCV that is resistant to boceprevir or telaprevir can occur if you take boceprevir or telaprevir alone, without peginterferon or ribavirin. Resistant HCV prevents you from clearing HCV from your body.

Preventing the development of HCV that is resistant to boceprevir and telaprevir is also important from the perspective of your future treatment. Boceprevir and telaprevir are the first generation of protease inhibitors, but many other potent inhibitors of the HCV protease are in clinical development. If you develop resistance to boceprevir or telaprevir, you may not respond to future treatments using similar inhibitors of the HCV NS3/4A protease.

WARNING: Patients with chronic HCV should *never* be treated with either telaprevir or boceprevir alone (monotherapy). Monotherapy is ineffective due to the rapid emergence of HCV variants resistant to the administered protease inhibitor. Viral variants resistant to one protease inhibitor may also be resistant to other protease inhibitors, including those currently being developed for future treatment.

AM I A CANDIDATE FOR TRIPLE THERAPY?

See Your Doctor and Get Evaluated. If you have chronic hepatitis C genotype 1 infection, you should be evaluated for triple therapy, whether you have never been treated (treatment-naïve) or have had prior treatment with interferon-based regimens (treatment-experienced). Triple therapy is effective to a greater or lesser degree in both treatment-naïve and treatment-experienced patients.

The drugs for treating HCV are powerful, and can have effects on many organs in your body beyond the liver. You may not be a candidate for interferon-based therapy if you have severe underlying conditions such as cardiac, pulmonary, neurologic, malignant, autoimmune, or infectious disease. Treatment may also be difficult if you have advanced liver disease or are a transplant recipient, dialysis patient, patient with HIV/HCV co-infection, or are a parent trying to get treatment for your child. In these cases, you should be treated by a provider with extensive experience, preferably in liver centers or specialized treatment units. If you have any of these conditions, your treatment provider may require more frequent laboratory testing and clinical assessments if triple therapy is initiated.

Interferon affects your mood, and the development of depression during treatment is common. If you have unstable or untreated psychiatric disease or are actively drinking alcohol or using drugs, you should seek treatment for these conditions prior to embarking on treatment for HCV.

Contraindications. The drugs comprising triple therapy are potent, and could potentially damage a developing fetus and cause birth defects. For this reason, you should not take triple therapy if you are pregnant, nursing, or trying to conceive. Double contraception (both man and woman) to avoid pregnancy is recommended during, and six months after, triple therapy for all couples of child-bearing potential.

Contraindications to peginterferon include an unstable psychiatric condition, serious underlying medical illness, active infection, or severe cytopenias. Contraindications to ribavirin include renal failure (ribavirin is cleared by the kidney), severe anemia, or any serious underlying skin condition. Contraindications to telaprevir or boceprevir include severe anemia. A serious underlying skin condition might also be a contraindication to telaprevir.

Telaprevir and boceprevir are metabolized by enzymes in the liver that also detoxify many other drugs or medications. Inform your physician or treatment provider whether you are taking any medications, over-the-counter products, or supplements. Your provider will need to determine which, if any, are allowable, and may need to consult a clinical pharmacist to check for significant interactions.

Triple Therapy Is Primarily for HCV Genotype 1 Infection. As indicated above, triple therapy is only currently approved for the treatment of HCV genotype 1 infection. Peginterferon with ribavirin is the mainstay of current therapy for the other HCV genotypes 2 through 6. Boceprevir and telaprevir were specifically designed to inhibit the NS3/4A protease of HCV genotype 1. Thus, triple therapy is uniquely appropriate for patients who are infected with HCV genotype 1.

There is very limited data regarding the effectiveness of telaprevir or boceprevir in the treatment of patients with non-1 genotypes of HCV. Existing studies suggest that telaprevir has activity against HCV genotype 2, but little activity against HCV genotype 3[80]. Currently, peginterferon plus ribavirin without boceprevir or telaprevir should be the initial treatment for non-1 genotypes of HCV.

Triple Therapy Is More Effective Than Peginterferon/Ribavirin in the Treatment of African Americans. If you are African American with HCV genotype 1 infection, triple therapy offers you an improved chance for cure over the previous treatment of peginterferon/ribavirin. You should consider evaluation and treatment with triple therapy.

What are your chances to achieve SVR and become cured? Past studies have indicated that African Americans were less responsive to interferon-based therapies. Peginterferon/ribavirin treatment yielded an SVR rate of only 25 percent in African Americans compared to 45 percent in Caucasian Americans.

The good news is that triple therapy improves your chance to achieve SVR (Figure 4B). In the boceprevir study of treatment-naïve patients (SPRINT-2), Black patients had SVR rates of 53 percent with triple therapy, compared to an SVR of 23 percent with peginterferon/ribavirin. In the telaprevir study of treatment-naïve patients (ILLUMINATE), the SVR of African Americans was 60 percent. These results indicate that

African Americans have a 50 to 60 percent chance for SVR with triple therapy—much higher than the 20 to 25 percent previously achieved with peginterferon/ribavirin.

FIGURE 4B: SVR IN AFRICAN AMERICANS IN TRIALS OF TRIPLE THERAPY: TREATMENT–NAÏVE PATIENTS

TELAPREVIR (ADVANCE)   BOCEPREVIR (SPRINT-2)

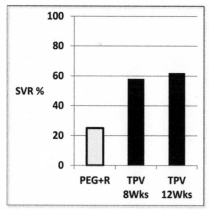 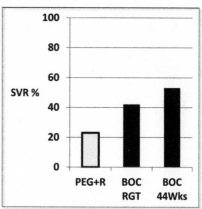

FIGURE 4B: Rates of SVR in African Americans enrolled into the trials of triple therapy are shown and compared to the results with peginterferon/ribavirin (PEG+R) given alone. Telaprevir (TPV) was given as for either eight (TPV 8Wks) or 12 (TPV 12Wks) weeks. Patients who had undetectable HCV RNA at weeks four and 12 received a total of 24 weeks of treatment. Boceprevir (BOC) was given as response guided therapy (BOC RGT) or as a fixed 44 week regimen (BOC 44 Wks). Patients who had undetectable HCV RNA at weeks eight and 24 received a total of 28 weeks of treatment. Triple therapy is more effective than peginterferon/ribavirin in African Americans.

Triple Therapy Is More Effective Than Peginterferon/Ribavirin in the Treatment of Patients with Advanced Fibrosis or Cirrhosis. Although noninvasive methods may emerge over the next few years, currently, the gold standard for defining the amount of scarring in your liver (fibrosis) is histologic evaluation of a liver biopsy. Pathologists assign stages to the amount of fibrosis as they examine your biopsy under the microscope. The most commonly used staging system is the Metavir Score, with stages ranging from 0 to 4. Stage 0 means no fibrosis, while stage 4 defines cirrhosis. Stages 1 through 3 are intermediate stages, with stage 1 indicating mild fibrosis, and stage 3 indicating more severe fibrosis with risk for evolution to cirrhosis. Some pathologists use a different system such as the Ishak Score, with stages ranging from 0 to 6. A score of 0 to 2 represents minimal fibrosis, 3 or 4 indicates moderate fibrosis, 5 is incomplete cirrhosis, and 6 is definite cirrhosis[34].

> *I have cirrhosis. My liver is badly damaged. Can triple therapy still work?*
>
> — *Connie*

The effectiveness of treatment is related to the severity of fibrosis. Patients with Metavir fibrosis stages 0 to 3 are more likely than patients with Metavir fibrosis stage 4 to clear HCV with antiviral treatment. This is true for both triple therapy and dual therapy with peginterferon/ribavirin, but the results with triple therapy in treatment-naïve patients are better at each stage of fibrosis. In the telaprevir trials of treatment-naïve patients, 76 percent of fibrosis stages 0-2, 65 percent of fibrosis stage 3, and 56 percent of fibrosis stage 4 treated with triple therapy achieved SVR. These results with triple therapy were far superior to those with peginterferon/ribavrin, where SVRs were only 47 percent, 36 percent, and 38 percent, respectively. With both treatments, patients with cirrhosis are less responsive, but at all stages of fibrosis, including cirrhosis, results are superior with triple therapy.

You are less likely to achieve SVR if you are treatment-experienced, and had either a partial or null response to PEGIFN/RBV (Figure 4C).

FIGURE 4C: FIBROSIS STAGE AND RESPONSIVENESS TO PEGINTERFERON/RIBAVIRIN DETERMINE LIKELIHOOD OF SVR WITH TELAPREVIR–BASED TRIPLE THERAPY

SVR (%)

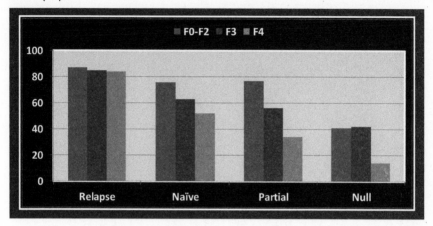

AASLD 2011. Pol S, et al. Hepatology 2011;54:374A.
CDDW/CASL 2012. Di Bisceglie A, et al. Can J Gastroenterol 2012;26: 81A.

FIGURE 4C: The impact of the stage of fibrosis and the severity of disease (X axis), and poor prior response to peginterferon/ribavirin (Prior Null) on SVR when treated with telaprevir-based triple therapy is shown. Best responders with the highest likelihood of achieving SVR are patients who relapsed or are naïve to prior treatment with minimal fibrosis. Poorest responders are null responders to peginterferon/ribavirin who have cirrhosis. "Comp cirrhosis" is compensated cirrhosis: biopsy evident cirrhosis, but without clinical or laboratory complications. "Decomp cirrhosis" is decompensated cirrhosis: either clinical or laboratory evidence of complications.

The decision to treat a patient with cirrhosis depends upon the clinical severity of their liver disease. Clinically, we define cirrhosis as either compensated or decompensated. If you have compensated cirrhosis (which implies that you have normal laboratory tests and no clinical manifestations of liver disease such as ascites, edema, varices, or encephalopathy), you can be treated. The registration trials for both boceprevir and telaprevir included a small percentage of patients with compensated cirrhosis. The FDA has recommended that patients with compensated cirrhosis who respond during triple therapy receive a full 48 weeks of treatment.

Decompensated cirrhosis implies advanced, clinically evident liver disease. If your doctor states that you have decompensated disease, this means that your laboratory tests are abnormal, your liver function is significantly impaired, and you have developed (or soon will develop) symptoms or clinical signs of liver disease. Some patients with decompensated cirrhosis can still be treated with antiviral therapy, but this should only be attempted in liver centers or in treatment centers with experience in HCV therapy and the management of patients with advanced liver disease.

MY DOCTOR TOLD ME THAT THE USE OF TRIPLE THERAPY IN MY CASE WOULD BE OFF LABEL. WHAT IS OFF LABEL?

The term "off label" refers to the use of a treatment for an indicator that is not yet approved by the FDA. Many patients with HCV have conditions that represent criteria for exclusion from participating in clinical trials of boceprevir or telaprevir. These special populations of patients have features that might alter management, influence virologic response, increase risk, worsen compliance or tolerability, and increase the cost of care. On the labels for boceprevir and telaprevir, these conditions are listed, and include non-1 HCV genotypes, decompensated cirrhosis, HIV/HCV co-infection, post-transplant status, and pediatric age. Use of triple therapy in these populations is, therefore, designated as "off label." Separate clinical studies or registration trials with the FDA would be required to shift from "off label" to "approved."

WARNING: Although the following discussion involves the "off-label" use of triple therapy, I am not endorsing widespread use of boceprevir or telaprevir in these populations. Nonetheless, care providers may determine that clinical necessity requires consideration of this treatment. The following discussion is meant to inform patients and their care providers of some of the key issues if triple therapy were to be considered.

USE OF TRIPLE THERAPY IF YOU ARE A PERSON WITH:
Non-1 HCV Genotypes

HCV Genotype 4. Only one clinical study has addressed triple therapy in HCV genotype 4 (presented at the European Association for the Study of the Liver meeting in April, 2011, by Y. Benhamou, et al, Abstract 828 [unpublished data]). In this study, 24 patients with HCV genotype 4 infections were evenly divided among three treatment Arms (also known as regimens or schedules). Patients in Arm 1 received two weeks of telaprevir monotherapy, followed by 46 weeks of peginterferon/ribavirin. Patients in Arm 2 received two weeks of telaprevir-based triple therapy, followed by 46 weeks of peginterferon/ribavirin. Lastly, patients in Arm 3 received 48 weeks of peginterferon/ribavirin. SVR rates were 63 percent, 50 percent, and 63 percent, respectively. Based on these findings, there was no significant effect of two weeks of telaprevir treatment on SVR in this very limited study.

Despite the lack of benefit of telaprevir in the study, two observations are noteworthy. First, the mean decline in HCV RNA during the two weeks of telaprevir monotherapy in Arm1 was only 0.77 $\log_{10}$, far less than the 4.77 $\log_{10}$ decline observed in a prior monotherapy study of HCV genotype 1. This finding suggests that patients infected with HCV genotype 4 are relatively unresponsive to telaprevir. On the other hand, the second finding of a more rapid rate of decline and greater reduction in HCV RNA in patients receiving triple therapy, compared to peginterferon/ribavirin, suggests a synergistic effect of telaprevir when added to peginterferon/ribavirin. Additional studies of HCV genotype 4, using 12 weeks of telaprevir-based triple therapy followed by 12 to 36 weeks of peginterferon/ribavirin, are needed to compare to the results achieved in patients with HCV genotype 1 infection.

HCV Genotype 2. Peginterferon/ribavirin without boceprevir or telaprevir is currently recommended for initial therapy of patients with non-1 genotypes, including HCV genotype 2 infection. The rate of clearing HCV genotype 2 with peginterferon/ribavirin exceeds 80 percent. The question is whether re-treatment using boceprevir or telaprevir added to peginterferon/ribavirin can be successful if you failed to clear HCV during a prior course of treatment with peginterferon/ribavirin. Unfortunately, clinical studies to answer this question have not yet been presented or published.

In the laboratory, investigators have used cell-based systems for measuring "in vitro" activity of antiviral agents against HCV, and have demonstrated that telaprevir has activity against non-1 genotypes, especially HCV genotype 2. Although clinical studies are limited[80], the laboratory replicon data (the lab system used for measuring the replication of the hepatitis C virus) provides at least a rationale for considering triple therapy for these patients.

Decompensated Cirrhosis

With decompensation, bilirubin and INR (prothrombin time) increase, and albumin and platelet count decrease. Clinical manifestations of decompensation include ascites, edema, varices, encephalopathy, easy bruisability, and bleeding. If you have decompensation, you may not tolerate the side effects of interferon-based therapy, and you could experience serious infection or further clinical deterioration with treatment.

Only 15 percent of patients with decompensated cirrhosis and HCV genotype 1 infection clear HCV when treated with peginterferon/ribavirin[60]. Triple therapy could possibly increase the rate of SVR. However, side effects and intolerability to peginterferon/ribavirin, boceprevir, or telaprevir are obstacles to the effectiveness of triple therapy in decompensated cirrhosis. Reductions in the doses of medications or discontinuation of any of the drugs used for triple therapy could reduce clearance of HCV and increase the risk for resistant HCV.

As noted above, if you have decompensated cirrhosis, and triple therapy is considered, you should only be evaluated and treated by providers experienced in the management of cirrhosis, advanced liver disease, and antiviral therapy. Ideally, this treatment should be administered in liver centers or highly experienced clinical units. Be advised that there are no published reports of either boceprevir or telaprevir in patients with decompensated liver disease. If available, you should consider enrollment in clinical trials specifically designed for patients with decompensated cirrhosis.

Liver Transplantation

My transplant in 2006 was for cirrhosis from HCV genotype 1. Now, the doctors say that the fibrosis in my transplanted liver is getting worse: fibrosis stage 3, almost cirrhosis. I'm worried that my liver is deteriorating, and I'll soon need a second transplant. Can I be treated with triple therapy?

— Fred

Studies of the use of triple therapy in transplant recipients are planned, and will likely start to enroll in 2012. Transplant centers have also developed their own treatment protocols for use with patients who are unable to enroll in the clinical trials. Given the experimental nature of triple therapy in this population of patients, whenever possible, it would be advisable to enroll post-transplant patients into clinical trials. However, many transplant recipients with recurrent HCV have progressive fibrosis, need urgent therapy, and will not have access to clinical trials.

There are several concerns in the treatment of post-transplant patients. Post-transplant patients are relatively resistant to interferon, and have high rates of viral replication and greater viral blood levels. Viral clearance using interferon or peginterferon plus ribavirin in HCV genotype 1 liver recipients is only 25 percent—surprisingly similar to the SVRs of other interferon-resistant groups such as African Americans and patients with cirrhosis. Interferon resistance may not only impair response to triple therapy, but may also increase the risk for viral resistance to boceprevir or telaprevir. A unique concern is immunosuppression may favor persistence of resistant HCV, which could lead to multi-drug resistance upon re-treatment with future direct-acting antiviral drugs.

Frequency and severity of anemia (low red cell count), low white blood cell count, and low platelet count during interferon-based therapy is much higher in transplant recipients. Treated liver recipients often require growth factors, such as erythropoietin analogue (EPO) and granulocyte colony stimulating factor (G-CSF). Anemia is potentially even more problematic with triple therapy. Treatment of anemia and low cell counts with growth factors greatly increases the cost of therapy, and EPO has safety concerns such as the risk of clotting and toxicity to the bone marrow, arresting production of red blood cells.

Tolerance to peginterferon/ribavirin is particularly poor in transplant recipients. Most require dose reductions in either or both drugs, and many will discontinue treatment altogether. Dose reductions or discontinuations of peginterferon or ribavirin will reduce the chances to clear HCV, and will increase the risk for viral resistance.

Finally, and perhaps most importantly, both boceprevir and telaprevir inhibit key metabolizing enzymes in the liver. Why is this important? The elimination or removal of several immunosuppressive medications (cyclosporine, tacrolimus, sirolimus, and everolimus) from the body is via metabolism in the liver. Administration of telaprevir or boceprevir will block the liver's metabolism of these immunosuppressive medications, blood levels will rise, and the risk for toxicity from the immunosuppressive drugs will increase[81].

Inhibition of a key liver enzyme by telaprevir is associated with a five-fold increase in cyclosporine exposure and a seventy-fold increase in tacrolimus exposure[82]. The reduction of doses and the frequency of dosing, along with religious monitoring of blood levels of immunosuppressive medication, would be essential. In addition, liver recipients who might take triple therapy need close clinical monitoring for toxicity, adverse events, and rejection. Optimal clinical management requires an experienced team including hepatologists, transplant coordinators, skilled nurses, and clinical pharmacologists.

Co-Infection with HIV and HCV

Clearly, the treatment of HCV co-infection in HIV patients represents an unmet medical need[83]. Current treatment with peginterferon/ribavirin is less effective in co-infected patients, and triple therapy promises to improve chances for SVR in these patients. Peginterferon/ribavirin treatment has yielded an SVR rate of only 25 percent in co-infected patients, compared to 45 percent in non-HIV cohorts. The good news is ongoing studies of triple therapy are demonstrating improved rates of on-treatment virologic response. Hopefully, the results of these studies to define the effectiveness of triple therapy for HIV/HCV co-infection will be available within the next 12 to 18 months.

One of the biggest issues in treatment of co-infected individuals is the potential for drug to drug interactions between boceprevir or telaprevir and the HIV prescription. Current clinical trials are being performed to study the use of an HIV prescription that minimizes the risk for adverse reactions with boceprevir or telaprevir.

A Child with Chronic HCV Infection

My son is now eleven years-old, he got his hepatitis C genotype 1 from me at the time of his birth. I was treated with peginterferon and ribavirin, and was cured. He was also treated similarly, and seemed to respond, since the virus disappeared from his blood during the treatment. But, after stopping treatment, the virus returned, he relapsed, and he now has fibrosis stage 2 to 3. I want to save my son from needing a liver transplant; how can I get him treatment?

— Lisa

Approvals of antiviral therapy for HCV in pediatric populations typically lag behind the dates of approvals in adults by several years. This raises a huge dilemma for the mother and child in the quote above: the child relapsed after a course of peginterferon/ribavirin, has significant fibrosis, and is now at risk for progression to cirrhosis. In addition, the child's prior experience indicates that he is a relapser, the type of response to peginterferon/ribavirin that is associated with the greatest likelihood to be cured by re-treatment with triple therapy. Yet, despite the need for triple therapy, and the anticipated likely success of this treatment, there is no availability due to the lack of studies and FDA approval. The only recourse is to refer the child to a pediatric liver center engaged in HCV treatment to see if a treatment protocol or clinical trial is available.

CAN YOU TEST MY BLOOD BEFORE TREATMENT TO SEE IF I WILL RESPOND TO TRIPLE THERAPY?

The single best pre-treatment predictor of achieving SVR in response to peginterferon/ribavirin is a polymorphism of the IL28b gene (encoding interferon lambda 3, which defines your response to interferon)[84]. Patients with the CC genotype of IL28b are more likely to spontaneously clear HCV after acute infection, and are more likely to clear HCV in response to peginterferon/ribavirin (60 to 70 percent) compared to CT or TT genotypes (20 to 30 percent). Other pre-treatment predictors of SVR are low viral load, lower BMI, non–African American race, and lower stage of fibrosis.

A similar (albeit less dramatic) effect of IL28b polymorphism in predicting the likelihood of SVR to triple therapy has also been observed (Figure 4D). In the telaprevir trials of treatment-naïve patients, the percentages of patients who cleared HCV were 90 percent for CC, 71 percent for CT, and 73 percent for TT IL28b genotypes[69, 71]. Results were very similar in the boceprevir trials: the percentage of patients who cleared HCV was 80 to 82 percent for CC, 65 to 71 percent for CT, and 55 to 59 percent for TT IL28b genotypes[68].

FIGURE 4D: SVR IN TRIALS OF TRIPLE THERAPY BY IL28B POLYMORPHISM TREATMENT-NAÏVE PATIENTS

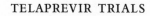

TELAPREVIR TRIALS

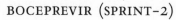

BOCEPREVIR (SPRINT-2)

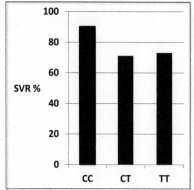

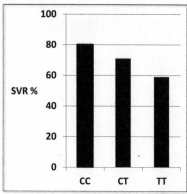

FIGURE 4D: The chance for SVR is excellent across all IL28B polymorphisms (genotypes CC, CT, or TT) with either telaprevir (left) or boceprevir (right) triple therapy.

The results from both the boceprevir and telaprevir trials indicate that response rates are high, even for patients with TT alleles. For this reason, the main value of the IL28b polymorphism in the setting of triple therapy is to provide information regarding the likelihood of response. Yet IL28b test results cannot be used to decide who to treat or who not to treat in regard to triple therapy.

· The best predictor of likelihood of HCV clearance during either peginterferon/ribavirin or triple therapy is the on-treatment response[85]. HCV RNA is measured monthly during the first several weeks of treatment. Patients who achieve undetectable HCV RNA within four weeks of triple therapy and continue to have undetectable HCV RNA while on therapy have about a 90 percent chance to be cured. This is true whether you are treated with peginterferon/ribavirin or triple therapy. Nonetheless, only 15 percent of patients treated with peginterferon/ribavirin, compared to 65 percent treated with telaprevir-based triple therapy, achieve rapid virologic response. Also, patients on triple therapy with rapid virologic response can achieve an SVR of about 90 percent with only six months of treatment required (see the section on "extended rapid virologic response" in chapter 5).

CONCLUDING REMARKS

My goal in this chapter has been to introduce you to some of the issues that determine whether you are a candidate for triple therapy. Like many newly emerging treatments, the clinical trials and research have not covered all the possible uses of the treatment, and further investigations are ongoing. For HCV genotype 1, the improvement in rates of clearance of HCV from 40 percent to over 70 percent represents a major step forward. Yet you might be infected with a different HCV genotype, or have clinical complications that would limit the effectiveness of this first generation of triple therapy based on boceprevir or telaprevir. Nonetheless, most patients with HCV genotype 1 infection should be considered for triple therapy, and those who qualify should anticipate an improvement in the chance for SVR. In chapter 5, I discuss the details of triple therapy and some of the unique nuances of treatment, monitoring, and follow-up, including discussion of the side effects and their management. In chapter 6, I speculate on the future of HCV therapy, based on the emerging results from early phase studies of new direct-acting and host-acting antiviral drugs. The new era is here—patients and providers should be excited.

5

TREATMENT WITH TRIPLE THERAPY

First Generation Inhibitors of the HCV NS3/4A Protease

I've had hepatitis C for years, and, for years, it was getting worse. My gastroenterologist suggested treatment. I searched the web for the results of triple therapy—I was surprised that nearly three of four treated patients were clearing hepatitis C. Very promising! I jumped on that and took peginterferon, ribavirin, and telaprevir. In four weeks, my blood was cleared of the hepatitis C virus: HCV RNA was undetectable. I was clear of hepatitis C on-treatment, and was able to stop after just six months. Unfortunately, I was one of the few with "eRVR" that relapse. Now, I am considering future treatment options.

Other persons with hepatitis C have asked me if they should try triple therapy. I tell them to go with triple therapy. There's more than a 70 percent chance that they will be cured if they take triple therapy. Those are good odds.

— Paul

TRIPLE THERAPY, the combination of peginterferon and ribavirin with either telaprevir or boceprevir, is the new standard of treatment for patients with chronic hepatitis C who are infected with HCV genotype 1. Triple therapy is superior to peginterferon/ribavirin in clearing HCV in both treatment-naïve[68, 69, 71] and treatment-experienced patients[67, 70].

This chapter focuses on issues related to treatment with triple therapy, including treatment effects, testing, clinical monitoring, side effects, and outcomes. One of my goals is to provide you with a roadmap to help you navigate your course as you journey forward in your quest to clear HCV with triple therapy. Hopefully, by reading this chapter, you will better understand how to determine if treatment is effective, and what to expect in terms of testing, side effects, and outcomes. The good news is triple therapy, when compared to peginterferon/ribavirin, will nearly double your chance of clearing HCV from your body.

In this chapter, I will discuss the following topics:

- What Exactly Is Triple Therapy?
  - Telaprevir-Based Triple Therapy
    — Telaprevir for Treatment-Naïve Patients
      - SVR
      - eRVR
      - Stop Guidelines
      - Treatment Algorithm
    — Telaprevir for Treatment-Experienced Patients
      - SVR
      - eRVR in Relapsers
      - Stop Guidelines
      - Treatment Algorithm
  - Boceprevir-Based Triple Therapy
    — Lead-In with Peginterferon and Ribavirin
    — Boceprevir for Treatment-Naïve Patients
      - SVR
      - eRVR'
      - Stop Guidelines
      - Treatment Algorithm

Telaprevir (INCIVEK®) and boceprevir (VICTRELIS®) were approved by the FDA for treatment of chronic hepatitis C in 2011. Although telaprevir and boceprevir were designed for HCV genotype 1, they have some activity against HCV genotypes 2 and 4. However, the clinical benefit of treating non-1 HCV genotypes with boceprevir or telaprevir has not yet been proven. Before you embark on a course of treatment, be sure to check your HCV genotype. Triple therapy is only FDA-approved for HCV genotype 1. Non-1 HCV genotypes are treated initially with peginterferon/ribavirin alone.

There are no randomized trials directly comparing boceprevir to telaprevir in terms of virologic response, safety, tolerability, and cost effectiveness. For this reason, I have purposefully avoided any direct comparison of these two treatments. In the sections on doses, formulations, tolerability, treatment algorithms, and side effects, I describe the information that is specific to either boceprevir or telaprevir[86].

Throughout this book and the following discussion, I use the term "triple therapy," which implies the use of peginterferon and ribavirin with boceprevir or telaprevir. When I use the term triple therapy alone, the information would apply to either boceprevir- or telaprevir-based treatment. When the information is specific to boceprevir or telaprevir, I use the terms boceprevir-based or telaprevir-based triple therapy.

In some circumstances, when making general statements or comments, I may use approximate values. On the other hand, when citing specific papers, I typically use the results as listed in the publication. Please refer to the list of references at the back of this book, which includes papers or other materials from which I have derived data to illustrate key points or focus the discussion. I encourage you to read the cited references, especially if you would like more detail regarding the results of specific studies.

The primary goal of therapy for chronic hepatitis C is to clear HCV from your body. We measure this clearance of HCV as sustained virologic response (SVR). This means that HCV RNA is not detected in your blood six months after the end of treatment. If you achieve SVR, you are very likely cured of HCV infection, because there is a less than 1 percent risk that your blood will, once again, become positive for HCV RNA.[77]

Today's treatment offers you a greater chance to be cured of HCV infection than ever before. The following sections describe in detail the use of triple therapy for chronic hepatitis C, the medications, and what you may expect for outcomes and side effects.

WHAT EXACTLY IS TRIPLE THERAPY?
Telaprevir-Based Triple Therapy

Telaprevir-based triple therapy is peginterferon, ribavirin, and telaprevir. All three drugs are required for maximum effectiveness. Rates of SVR are lower if either peginterferon or ribavirin is removed from the treatment regimen[87].

> I was excited to be in the study. I was assigned to a treatment arm that excluded ribavirin, which can be really hard on your body. I only had to take the peginterferon and telaprevir. However, at week six of treatment, while I was vacationing in Fort Lauderdale with a friend, I got an urgent

call from my nurse, "Stop the drugs, the virus broke through!" I was paralyzed by the news. My hopes had been running high that I would be cured—maybe if I had had the ribavirin, I would be cured. All of the patients I knew who took all three drugs were virus-free. My doctors and nurses are discussing how best to re-treat me, now or in the future. I'm sure I'll have options, likely with ribavirin in the mix.

— *Carol*

Telaprevir-based triple therapy is effective in both treatment-naïve and treatment-experienced patients[69, 70, 71]. Treatment-naïve patients or patients who have relapsed after PEGIFN/RBV with rapid and sustained clearance of HCV RNA may be able to stop treatment after 24 weeks. Other patients who respond more slowly should be treated for 48 weeks to achieve best results.

If you choose telaprevir-based triple therapy, you will start your treatment with 12 weeks of telaprevir in combination with peginterferon and ribavirin. After 12 weeks, you will stop telaprevir, but continue your treatment with either 12 or 36 additional weeks of peginterferon and ribavirin. Your total treatment could be as short as 24 weeks or as long as 48 weeks.

Here are the three main factors that will determine whether you can stop after only 24 weeks of treatment:

1. The speed with which the HCV RNA drops or declines in your blood after starting treatment,
2. Whether or not you have cirrhosis, and
3. The category of response during a prior course of treatment.

Telaprevir for Treatment-Naïve Patients. The phase III trials that established the effectiveness of telaprevir-based triple therapy for treatment-naïve patients were ADVANCE[71] and ILLUMINATE[69] (Figure 5A). The primary data from these trials were submitted to the FDA for final approval of telaprevir in treating chronic hepatitis C.

FIGURE 5A: SVR IN TREATMENT–NAÏVE PATIENTS

(% WITH SVR)

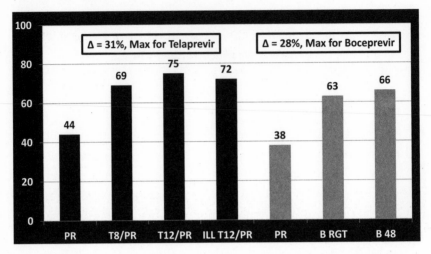

ADVANCE. N Engl J Med 2011;364:2405-2416. ILLUMINATE. N Engl J Med 2011;365:1014-1024. SPRINT-2. N Engl J Med 2011;364:1195-1206.

FIGURE 5A: Rates of SVR with triple therapy in treatment-naïve patients is shown for telaprevir (black bars) and boceprevir (gray bars). With both treatments, there is approximately a 30 percent improvement in the chance for SVR with peginterferon/ribavirin alone. PR, peginterferon/ribavirin; T8/PR, eight-week telaprevir regimen; T12/PR, 12-week telaprevir regimen; ILL T12/PR, result from ILLUMINATE trial; B RGT, boceprevir using response guided therapy; B 48, boceprevir using a fixed total 48 week regimen (44 weeks of boceprevir).

SVR. With telaprevir-based triple therapy, you have approximately three chances out of four to clear HCV and achieve a sustained virologic response (SVR). SVR is defined as undetectable HCV RNA six months or more after the end of treatment. In the FDA analyses, the rates of SVR were 79 percent in ADVANCE and 74 percent in ILLUMINATE—an increase in SVR of 33 percent over the previous standard of care, peginterferon/ribavirin. When you achieve SVR, you are likely cured of HCV infection: you will have less than a 1 percent chance that the HCV infection will return in future years of follow-up. With triple therapy, you have an excellent chance to be cured of your HCV genotype 1 infection.

PUBLISHED RATES OF SVR IN TREATMENT–NAÏVE PATIENTS TREATED WITH TELAPREVIR

Clinical Trial	% SVR
ADVANCE	75%
ILLUMINATE	72%

These rates of SVR are a striking improvement over the 42 percent achieved with peginterferon/ribavirin.

Mentally, I was ready to do whatever was necessary to beat hepatitis C. Although I had never previously been treated, I was ready for triple therapy. However, once I was on treatment, I realized that there was more to endure than taking the medicines at exactly the prescribed times. First and foremost, I had to commit myself to succeed. The side effects of dry skin and other skin-related issues, and the need to scratch upon every door jam, was a constant thought. I invested part of my life-savings in creams and lotions. Secondly, I committed to abstinence—no alcohol, not even a beer at dinner. Mental toughness was the key to getting through each day. During treatment, I battled mental and physical hard-ships, but seeing the results indicating that HCV RNA was no longer detected in my blood did wonders to maintain a positive outlook. I truly believed that if I persevered through the entire course of treatment, cure would be my reward at the end. Commitment and perseverance carried me through. Now, three years later, I'm cured: the tests for HCV RNA remain negative. Obviously, I have no regrets that I elected treatment.

— Mark

The treatment of my hepatitis C in that clinical trial is best described as the worst case of flu I ever had. But, now, I'm over it: no hepatitis C!

— *Terry*

eRVR. Because triple therapy is much more potent than peginterferon/ribavirin, your chance to clear HCV and achieve SVR is nearly double that observed with peginterferon/ribavirin. In addition, the rate of decline in HCV RNA is much faster with triple therapy: the HCV RNA in your blood may become undetectable as soon as one or two weeks after beginning treatment. This rapid and persistent decline in HCV RNA requires a new definition, extended rapid virologic response (eRVR). Extended rapid virologic response (eRVR) is defined as clearance of HCV RNA by week four of treatment and the persistence of undetectable HCV RNA throughout the remainder of the first 12 weeks of telaprevir-based triple therapy. If you achieve eRVR, you have a great chance to be cured of HCV.

In the ILLUMINATE trial, 65 percent of patients achieved eRVR, and more than 90 percent of the patients with eRVR achieved SVR. In addition, this study also demonstrated that there was no advantage to extending the treatment beyond 24 weeks in the patients who achieved eRVR.

- **The Significance of eRVR:** What does all of this mean to you? Here is the bottom line: if you achieve eRVR, you will only need 24 weeks of treatment, and can expect a 90 percent chance to be cured of HCV.

- **Cirrhosis.** Cirrhosis is an exception when applying the eRVR rule of stopping therapy at 24 weeks. If you have cirrhosis, you will have greater difficulty in clearing HCV and achieving SVR, even if you experience eRVR. Cirrhosis is a condition that is relatively resistant to antiviral treatment, so if you have cirrhosis and have managed to achieve eRVR, it is recommended that you extend the PEGIFN/ RBV period of treatment for a total of 48 weeks.

Stop Guidelines. Although triple therapy is highly effective in most cases, in some cases, the treatment fails to clear HCV. Early changes in HCV RNA during treatment predict your likelihood of achieving SVR. Poor response and inability to achieve SVR is defined by HCV RNA:

1. Greater than 1000 IU/mL at treatment week four, or
2. Greater than 1000 IU/mL at treatment week 12, or
3. Positive at week 24.

If you meet any of these criteria, you will not achieve SVR, and it is recommended that you stop all treatment medications. You must also stop treatment if HCV RNA rebounds while taking telaprevir, as this can represent the emergence of HCV variants resistant to telaprevir.

> *Unfortunately, I was one of the non-responders. My viral count started to fall immediately on triple therapy, but, around week six, it started to increase. My doctor told me that the virus was developing resistance, so I had to stop the treatment. I have lived with hepatitis C for 10 years; I was hoping that triple therapy would beat it. Now, I'm reading articles and watching the Internet for new developments: there are a lot of new drugs and treatments in trials.*
>
> — *Gary*

Treatment Algorithm. Figure 5B is the treatment algorithm that you should review if you have decided on telaprevir-based triple therapy, and you have never previously been treated for chronic hepatitis C.

FIGURE 5B: TELAPREVIR ALGORITHM FOR
TREATMENT–NAÏVE PATIENTS

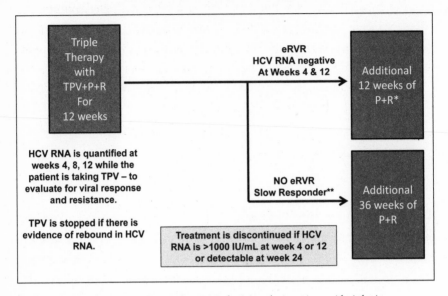

* FDA recommends extending P+R for 36 weeks in patients with cirrhosis.

** Slow responder is RNA positive at week 4 but RNA negative prior to or at week 24.

FIGURE 5B: Algorithm for telaprevir (TPV)-based therapy of chronic hepatitis C in treatment-naïve patients with genotype 1 infection based on results from the ADVANCE and ILLUMINATE trials. Treatment is initiated with TPV plus peginterferon (P) and ribavirin (R), and HCV RNA is measured monthly during the first three months. TPV is stopped at week 12 and eRVR (negative HCV RNA at weeks four and 12) is determined. In the ILLUMINATE trial, 65 percent of patients experienced eRVR. Patients with eRVR are treated for an additional 12 weeks of P+R. Patients with cirrhosis and eRVR should be treated with an additional 36 weeks of P+R (as recommended by the FDA). Patients without eRVR, but who achieved HCV RNA <1000 IU/mL at weeks four and 12 and are HCV RNA negative at week 24, are treated for an additional 36 weeks with P+R. Treatment is stopped if HCV RNA is >1000 IU/mL at week four or 12 or positive at week 24.

- *eRVR.* Treatment is initiated with 12 weeks of telaprevir (TPV), peginterferon (P), and ribavirin (R). Telaprevir is always given for only 12 weeks. If you achieve eRVR, you will complete your course of treatment with an additional 12 weeks of peginterferon/ribavirin. If you have cirrhosis, you will complete treatment with an additional 36 weeks of peginterferon/ribavirin, even if you achieve eRVR.
- *Slow Responder.* Slow responders have detectable HCV RNA at week four, but undetectable HCV RNA by week 24. If you are a slow responder, you will receive an additional 36 weeks of peginterferon/ribavirin.

As stated above, treatment is discontinued if HCV RNA is greater than 1000 IU/mL at weeks four or 12, or if it is positive at week 24.

Telaprevir for Treatment-Experienced Patients. If you previously received a course of peginterferon/ribavirin, but still have chronic hepatitis C, you are classified as treatment-experienced. Your type of prior treatment experience is further categorized as null, partial, breakthrough, or relapse, based upon HCV RNA measurements during and after the course of the prior treatment[50].

- **Null:** Null response is defined as less than a ten-fold decrease ($<1\log_{10}$ IU/mL) in HCV RNA by week four or less than a 100-fold decrease ($<2\log_{10}$ IU/mL) by week 12 during a prior course of peginterferon/ribavirin.
- **Partial:** Partial response is defined as greater than a 100-fold decrease ($>2\log_{10}$ IU/mL) in HCV RNA by week 12, but a persistently positive HCV RNA throughout prior treatment.
- **Breakthrough:** Breakthrough is defined as an emergence of a positive HCV RNA after achieving undetectable HCV RNA while on prior treatment. Breakthrough is usually a result of a decrease in dose or missed dose(s) of antiviral medication.
- **Relapse:** Relapse is defined by an undetectable HCV RNA at the end of prior treatment, but positive HCV RNA during follow-up.

These categories of response, from null to partial to breakthrough/relapse, reflect increasing sensitivity to interferon (Figure 5C). Clearing HCV RNA from your blood during a prior course of peginterferon/ribavirin suggests that you respond well to interferon. If you are a relapse, you are quite sensitive to interferon, and are very likely to achieve SVR when re-treated with triple therapy.

FIGURE 5C: SVR IN TREATMENT–EXPERIENCED PATIENTS (% WITH SVR)

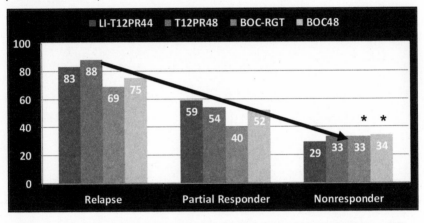

Zeuzem S, et al. REALIZE final results. N Engl J Med 2011;364:2417-2428. Bacon BR, et al. RESPOND-2 final results. N Engl J Med 2011;364:1207-1217.

FIGURE 5C: The results of triple therapy when used to re-treat patients whose prior treatment was peginterferon/ribavirin. See text for definitions of prior treatment response. Relapsers have the best response when re-treated with triple therapy. LI-T12PR48, four weeks of peginterferon/ribavirin as Lead-In (LI) plus 12 weeks of telaprevir plus total of 48 weeks of peginterferon/ribavirin; T12PR48, 12 weeks of telaprevir plus 48 weeks of peginterferon/ribavirin; BOC-RGT, response-guided boceprevir; BOC48, fixed 48-week boceprevir regimen.

SVR. The FDA approved telaprevir-based triple therapy for treatment-experienced patients, based upon the results of the REALIZE trial[70]. All patients in this trial were targeted to receive a total of 48 weeks of treatment. Shortening treatment duration based on eRVR was not evaluated.

If you have previously been treated with peginterferon/ribavirin, and desire to be treated with telaprevir-based triple therapy, you may ask, "What are my chances for cure?" The key to answering this question is the category of virologic response that you experienced during the prior course of peginterferon/ribavirin. Your chance to be cured by re-treatment with telaprevir-based triple therapy, based upon your prior treatment response, is shown in the following table.

SVR IN TREATMENT–EXPERIENCED PATIENTS RE–TREATED WITH TELAPREVIR

Prior Response to PEGIFN/RBV	% SVR, Re-treatment
Relapse	88%
Partial Response	59%
Null Response	30%

For comparison, if you are re-treated with another course of peginterferon/ribavirin without telaprevir, your chances for SVR are only 24 percent for prior relapse, 15 percent for partial response, and 5 percent for null response. So, despite the failure of prior treatment with peginterferon/ribavirin to clear your HCV, re-treatment with telaprevir-based triple therapy can be successful. Re-treatment is especially effective if you have relapsed or had a partial response during your prior course of peginterferon/ribavirin. Triple therapy is not as effective if you have had a null response to prior peginterferon/ribavirin.

Given that this was my fourth course of treatment, I pretty much knew what to expect—or so I thought. This treatment was the toughest of them all. Although the rash wasn't too bad, the fatigue was worse. I would

*come home from work, sit in front of the TV and stare for three hours,
then get up from the couch and go to bed. While I was on this treatment,
I was working in two different states, and had to fly on a weekly basis.
I was cold all the time, and, out of necessity, carried my "blankey" with
me at all times. Unfortunately, it was blue, and a flight attendant asked
me to refrain from taking the plane's blanket upon disembarking. I wore
a sweatshirt in June, and I live in the southwest: a hot place, generally.*

*Despite the trials and tribulations, I persisted and continued the
treatment. I'm glad I did, as the tests indicate that the hepatitis C is
gone. It's been two years, and my HCV RNA remains negative; despite
the challenges, it was worth it.*

— Barb

eRVR in Relapsers. Extended rapid virologic response (eRVR) was not
evaluated in the REALIZE trial. Nonetheless, the FDA recommends
that a prior relapser who achieves eRVR during re-treatment with
telaprevir-based triple therapy can stop treatmen at week 24. All other
treatment-experienced patients who are responding to re-treatmen to
triple therapy should receive 48 weeks of treatment.

Stop Guidelines. Not all patients respond to triple therapy. Indicators of
poor response and an inability to achieve SVR are HCV RNA:

1. Greater than 1000 IU/mL at treatment week four, or
2. Greater than 1000 IU/mL at treatment week 12, or
3. Positive at week 24.

If you meet any of these criteria, you will not clear HCV, and it is
recommended that you stop all treatment medications. Also, you must
stop treatment if HCV RNA rebounds while taking telaprevir, as this
can represent the emergence of HCV variants resistant to telaprevir.

Even though I relapsed after the telaprevir treatment, I have a lot more energy than I had before the treatment. I think giving my liver a break for a few months by being free of the virus helped to contribute to my new-found energy.

— *Paul*

Treatment Algorithm. Figure 5D is the treatment algorithm that you should review if you have decided on telaprevir-based triple therapy, and you have had a prior course of peginterferon/ribavirin.

FIGURE 5D: TELAPREVIR ALGORITHM FOR TREATMENT–EXPERIENCED PATIENTS

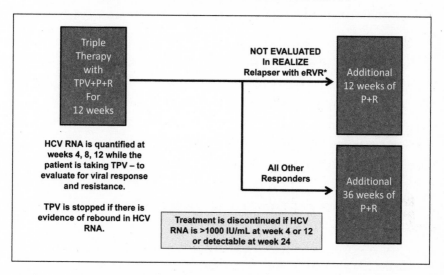

* *FDA indicates that relapsers (during prior course of PEG/RBV) who achieve eRVR can stop at week 24.*

FIGURE 5D: Algorithm for telaprevir (TPV)-based therapy of chronic hepatitis C in treatment-experienced patients with genotype 1 infection based on results from the REALIZE trial. All patients responding to the regimen (HCV RNA <1000 IU/mL at weeks four and 12 and HCV RNA negative at week 24), regardless of eRVR, receive 36 weeks of P+R. The FDA has indicated that prior relapsers achieving eRVR only need 12 additional weeks of P+R. Treatment is stopped if HCV RNA is >1000 IU/mL at week four or 12 or positive at week 24.

You will initiate treatment with 12 weeks of telaprevir (TPV), peginterferon (P), and ribavirin (R). If you had relapsed after a prior course of peginterferon/ribavirin, and now have achieved eRVR during retreatment with telaprevir-based triple therapy, you only need an additional 12 weeks of peginterferon/ribavirin.

If you had any other category of prior response (or have cirrhosis), and respond to telaprevir-based triple therapy, you should receive an additional 36 weeks of peginterferon/ribavirin, regardless of eRVR. Treatment is discontinued if HCV RNA is greater than 1000 IU/mL at weeks four or 12 or if it is positive at week 24.

Boceprevir-Based Triple Therapy

Boceprevir-based triple therapy is effective in both treatment-naïve and treatment-experienced patients[67, 68]. Treatment-naïve patients without cirrhosis who clear HCV by week eight of treatment may be able to stop treatment at week 28. Treatment-experienced patients who lack cirrhosis and clear HCV RNA by week eight may be able to stop treatment at week 36.

If you choose to be treated with boceprevir-based triple therapy, your treatment will begin with a four week lead-in with peginterferon/ribavirin. After this lead-in, your subsequent treatment with boceprevir plus peginterferon/ribavirin will be for 24, 32, or 44 weeks. The factors that determine your total duration of treatment are:

- The amount of decline in HCV RNA during lead-in,
- The rate of decline in HCV RNA during the first 20 weeks of boceprevir/peginterferon/ribavirin,
- Whether you have cirrhosis, and,
- If you are treatment-experienced, the type of response that you had during your prior course with peginterferon and ribavirin.

Lead-In with Peginterferon and Ribavirin. A unique feature of boceprevir-based triple therapy is a four week lead-in (LI) with peginterferon/ribavirin prior to starting boceprevir. Lead-in does not seem to increase your chance to achieve SVR, or decrease your risk to develop HCV variants that are resistant to treatment. Lead-in, however, does define your responsiveness to interferon. If you experience a ten-fold ($>1\log_{10}$ IU/mL) or greater decrease in HCV RNA during lead-in, you are more likely to achieve SVR compared to patients in whom HCV RNA declines less.

Boceprevir for Treatment-Naïve Patients.

SVR. The SPRINT-2 trial was the basis for FDA approval of boceprevir-based triple therapy for treatment-naïve patients[68] (Figure 5A). Two groups of patients were studied: black and non-black. Because of the multinational nature of SPRINT-2, black patients were not solely African Americans: some were European of African descent. In black patients, boceprevir-based triple therapy achieved SVRs of 42 percent to 53 percent, compared to an SVR of only 23 percent with peginterferon/ribavirin. In non-black patients, boceprevir-based triple therapy achieved SVRs of 67 percent to 68 percent, compared to an SVR of 40 percent with peginterferon/ribavirin. In both black and non-black populations, boceprevir-based triple therapy was superior to peginterferon/ribavirin.

SVR IN TREATMENT–NAÏVE PATIENTS TREATED
WITH BOCEPREVIR

Patient Groups in SPRINT-2	% SVR
Non-Black	67%, 68%
Black	42%, 53%

Your ability to achieve SVR in response to boceprevir-based triple therapy is also predicted by the decline in HCV RNA during lead-in. The chance of achieving SVR is over 80 percent if you achieve at least a ten-fold ($>1\log_{10}$ IU/mL) decline in HCV RNA during lead-in. The link between SVR and the decline in HCV RNA during lead-in emphasizes the importance of your ability to respond to interferon in determining the success of your treatment.

eRVR'. In the boceprevir trials, extended rapid virologic response (eRVR') was defined as undetectable HCV RNA from treatment weeks eight through 24. In the SPRINT-2 trial, 44 percent of patients achieved eRVR', and were eligible to stop treatment at week 28 (four weeks of lead-in plus 24 weeks of boceprevir, peginterferon, and ribavirin). If you have cirrhosis, or if your HCV RNA fails to decline during the four weeks of lead-in, the FDA has recommended that you receive 44 weeks total of boceprevir-based triple therapy, even if you experience eRVR'.

Stop Guidelines. As with telaprevir, triple therapy with boceprevir fails to clear HCV in some cases. Indicators of poor response and inability to achieve SVR are HCV RNA:

1. Greater than 100 IU/mL at treatment week twelve, or
2. Positive at week 24.

If either of these criteria is met, you cannot clear HCV, will not achieve SVR, and your treatment should be discontinued. Also, you must stop treatment if HCV RNA rebounds while taking boceprevir, as this can represent the emergence of HCV variants resistant to boceprevir.

Treatment Algorithm. Figure 5E is the treatment algorithm that you should review if you have decided on boceprevir-based triple therapy, and you have not been previously treated with peginterferon/ribavirin.

FIGURE 5E: BOCEPREVIR ALGORITHM
FOR TREATMENT–NAÏVE PATIENTS

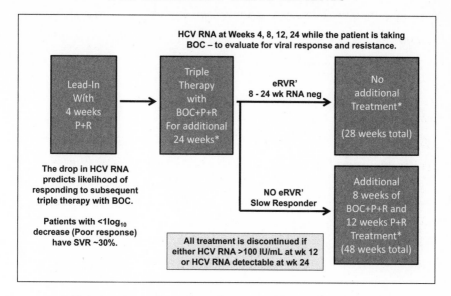

HCV RNA at Weeks 4, 8, 12, 24 while the patient is taking BOC – to evaluate for viral response and resistance.

Lead-In With 4 weeks P+R → Triple Therapy with BOC+P+R For additional 24 weeks*

eRVR' 8 - 24 wk RNA neg → No additional Treatment* (28 weeks total)

NO eRVR' Slow Responder → Additional 8 weeks of BOC+P+R and 12 weeks P+R Treatment* (48 weeks total)

The drop in HCV RNA predicts likelihood of responding to subsequent triple therapy with BOC.

Patients with <1log$_{10}$ decrease (Poor response) have SVR ~30%.

All treatment is discontinued if either HCV RNA >100 IU/mL at wk 12 or HCV RNA detectable at wk 24

* *Cirrhotic patients and Poor Responders are treated for 44 weeks BOC+P+R, regardless of eRVR'.*

** *Slow responders are RNA positive at week 8 but RNA negative prior to or at week 24.*

FIGURE 5E: Algorithm for boceprevir (BOC)-based therapy of chronic hepatitis C in treatment-naïve patients with genotype 1 infection based on results from the SPRINT-2 trial. Treatment is initiated with a four-week lead-in period of peginterferon (P) plus ribavirin (R). After lead-in, BOC plus P+R is initiated and continued while HCV RNA is measured at weeks four, eight, 12, and 24. If HCV RNA is negative from weeks eight through 24 (eRVR: approximately 45 percent of patients), then all treatment is stopped at week 28. If HCV RNA is positive between weeks eight to 24 but negative at week 24, then BOC plus P+R is continued for an additional eight weeks, followed by an additional 12 weeks of P+R (per FDA guidelines). Patients with cirrhosis or poor response during lead-in (<1log$_{10}$ decline in HCV RNA) receive BOC plus P+R for 44 weeks (per FDA guidelines). Treatment is stopped if HCV RNA is >100 IU/mL at week 12 or positive at week 24.

Treatment is initiated with a four week lead-in of peginterferon/ribavirin (P+R), and followed by 24 weeks of boceprevir (BOC), peginterferon (P), and ribavirin (R). If you do not have cirrhosis, you may be able to stop treatment at week 28 if you experience:

- At least a $1\log_{10}$ IU/mL (ten-fold) decline in HCV RNA during lead-in, and
- Achieve eRVR'.

If you have cirrhosis or do not meet the criteria to stop at week 28, a longer duration of treatment is necessary. The durations vary depending upon presence or absence of cirrhosis, drop in HCV RNA during lead-in, or rate of decline on boceprevir-based triple therapy.

- **Cirrhosis.** If you have cirrhosis, but you still achieve negative HCV RNA by treatment week 24, you will receive 20 additional weeks of boceprevir/peginterferon/ribavirin, for a total treatment of 48 weeks (four weeks lead-in, 44 weeks boceprevir/peginterferon/ribavirin).
- **Minimal Drop in HCV RNA During Lead-In.** If HCV RNA fails to decline at least ten-fold ($1\log_{10}$ IU/mL) during lead-in, but you still achieve negative HCV RNA by treatment week 24, you will receive 20 additional weeks of boceprevir/peginterferon/ribavirin, for a total treatment of 48 weeks (four weeks lead-in, 44 weeks boceprevir/peginterferon/ribavirin).
- **Slow Responders.** If HCV RNA declines to less than 100 IU/mL, but is still detectable at week 12, and then becomes undetectable by week 24, you will receive an additional eight weeks of boceprevir/peginterferon/ribavirin, followed by 12 additional weeks of peginterferon and ribavirin (four weeks lead-in, 32 weeks boceprevir/peginterferon/ribavirin, 12 weeks peginterferon/ribavirin).

Boceprevir for Treatment-Experienced Patients
The definitions of various categories of treatment-experienced patients

are given on page 93. You may find it helpful to review these categories and their definitions before reading the following section.

SVR. The RESPOND-2 trial was the basis for FDA approval of boceprevir-based triple therapy for treatment-experienced patients[67] (Figure 5C). The patients who enrolled in RESPOND-2 were either partial responders or relapsers; null responders were not enrolled. A second trial, PROVIDE, has studied null responders. Overall, in RESPOND-2, the rates of SVR ranged from 59 percent to 67 percent for boceprevir-based triple therapy. These results were superior to the SVR of only 21 percent in the patients re-treated with peginterferon/ribavirin.

Factors that improve your chance to achieve SVR are:

1. HCV RNA decline during a prior course of peginterferon/ribavirin,
2. HCV RNA decline during lead-in, and
3. Absence of cirrhosis.

- **Relapsers.** If you have relapsed after a prior course of peginterferon/ribavirin, you have an excellent chance to be cured by re-treatment with triple therapy. Based upon the results in RESPOND-2, your likelihood of achieving SVR by re-treatment would be 69 percent to 75 percent.

- **Partial Responders.** If you had a partial response during a prior course of peginterferon/ribavirin, the level of HCV RNA declined in your blood by at least $2\log_{10}$ IU/mL (100-fold), but was never undetectable. You would have a very good chance to be cured by re-treatment with triple therapy. Based upon the results in RESPOND-2, your likelihood of achieving SVR by re-treatment would be 40 percent to 52 percent.

- **Null Responders.** Null response, defined by less than 100-fold ($<2\log_{10}$ IU/mL) drop in HCV RNA during peginterferon/

ribavirin, implies that you are poorly responsive to interferon. Based on the results from PROVIDE (presented at the American Association for the Study of Liver Diseases meeting, November, 2011), your likelihood of achieving SVR by re-treatment with boceprevir-based triple therapy is 37 percent.

- **Decrease in HCV RNA During Lead-In.** The decrease in HCV RNA during the lead-in period of peginterferon/ribavirin also predicts your likelihood of achieving SVR. If you experience greater than a $1\log_{10}$ IU/mL drop (more than ten-fold drop) in HCV RNA, your chance for SVR is 73 percent to 80 percent. In contrast, if you experience less than a $1\log_{10}$ IU/mL drop (less than ten-fold drop) in HCV RNA, your chance for SVR is 33 percent to 34 percent.

- **Cirrhosis.** Generally, if you have cirrhosis, you are less likely to achieve SVR with triple therapy. The results from RESPOND-2 suggest that, if you have cirrhosis, your chance for SVR might be higher if boceprevir-based triple therapy is extended for 44 weeks.

Stop Guidelines. Under certain circumstances, boceprevir-based triple therapy will not result in SVR, and continuing treatment would be futile. If your blood tests indicate either of the following, you will not achieve SVR:

1. HCV RNA is greater than 100 IU/mL at treatment week 12, or
2. HCV RNA is positive at week 24

If either of these criteria is met, you should discontinue all treatment medications. You must also stop treatment if HCV RNA rebounds while taking boceprevir, as this can represent the emergence of HCV variants resistant to boceprevir.

Treatment Algorithm. Figure 5F is the treatment algorithm that you should review if you have decided on boceprevir-based triple therapy, and you have had a prior course of peginterferon/ribavirin.

FIGURE 5F: BOCEPREVIR ALGORITHM
FOR TREATMENT–EXPERIENCED PATIENTS

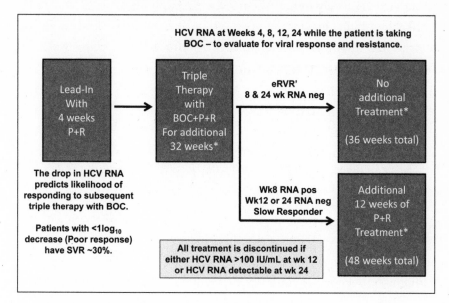

HCV RNA at Weeks 4, 8, 12, 24 while the patient is taking BOC – to evaluate for viral response and resistance.

Lead-In With 4 weeks P+R

The drop in HCV RNA predicts likelihood of responding to subsequent triple therapy with BOC.

Patients with <$1\log_{10}$ decrease (Poor response) have SVR ~30%.

Triple Therapy with BOC+P+R For additional 32 weeks*

eRVR'
8 & 24 wk RNA neg

No additional Treatment*
(36 weeks total)

Wk8 RNA pos
Wk12 or 24 RNA neg
Slow Responder

Additional 12 weeks of P+R Treatment*
(48 weeks total)

All treatment is discontinued if either HCV RNA >100 IU/mL at wk 12 or HCV RNA detectable at wk 24

Patients with Cirrhosis, Prior Null Response, or Poor Response are considered for 44 weeks of BOC+P+R, regardless of eRVR'.

FIGURE 5F: Algorithm for boceprevir (BOC)-based therapy of chronic hepatitis C in treatment-experienced patients with genotype 1 infection based on results from the RESPOND-2 trial. The algorithm is similar to that shown in Figure 5C, except that, with response-guided BOC plus P+R, triple therapy is given for 32 weeks. If HCV RNA is negative from weeks eight through 24, then all treatment is stopped at week 36. If HCV RNA is positive at week eight, but negative at week 24, then P+R is continued for an additional 12 weeks. Patients with cirrhosis, prior null response, or poor response during lead-in are treated with BOC plus P+R for 44 weeks (per FDA guidelines). Treatment is stopped if HCV RNA is >100 IU/mL at week 12 or positive at week 24.

You will be treated with a four week lead-in of peginterferon/ribavirin (P+R), and then 32 weeks of boceprevir/peginterferon/rivavirin (BOC+P+R). If you do not have cirrhosis, and HCV RNA is undetectable at weeks eight through 24, your treatment will stop at week

36. If your tests detect HCV RNA at earlier timepoints, but HCV RNA is undetectable at week 24, you will receive 12 additional weeks of peginterferon/ribavirin. If you have cirrhosis, experience less than a ten-fold ($<1\log_{10}$ IU/mL) drop in HCV RNA during lead-in, or are a prior null responder to PEGIFN/RBV, you will receive 44 weeks of boceprevir/peginterferon/ribavirin.

SIDE EFFECTS OF TRIPLE THERAPY

The side effects are fun, fun, fun. I have flu-like symptoms, extreme fatigue, rashes, and anemia. I count the days, months, and weeks, and every time my blood is tested and is still clear, it gives me hope. I have a family who supports me, and my work supports me.

— Carl

You may experience side effects from any or all of the drugs in the triple therapy regimen.

WARNING: Do not reduce doses or skip doses of telaprevir or boceprevir. The doses of telaprevir or boceprevir should never be reduced, due to the risk of the emergence of viral resistance to these and related protease inhibitors. When side effects cannot be managed by other strategies, it may be necessary to discontinue telaprevir or boceprevir. In a patient with virologic response who discontinues telaprevir or boceprevir due to side effects, peginterferon/ribavirin may still be continued.

Peginterferon and Ribavirin

Peginterferon side effects include flu-like symptoms, mood disorder, depression, cytopenias (lowering of white blood cells, red blood cells [anemia], and platelets), and risk for infection. Ribavirin side effects include breakdown of red blood cells (hemolytic anemia), rash, and the worsening of peginterferon side effects. Other rare reactions can include pulmonary, renal, cardiac, and neurologic illnesses, and exacerbation of underlying conditions such as autoimmune disease, thyroid disease, arthritic conditions, and dermatologic conditions.

I mostly have fatigue. I try to stay rested and hydrated. The fatigue is mainly from the interferon. I take a shot Monday morning, and, by the evening, I just feel lousy. By Wednesday, I begin to feel better, again. Those two interferon days are rough, but I know the side effects will pass.

Sex drive and function goes away when you are on these drugs, but not entirely. I still have a sex-life, just not as often. It's part of the game, and it will all get better when I'm done with the treatment.

— Allen

Treatment has affected my personal relationships in terms of intimacy. I'm waiting for treatment to be over. The sex drive comes back; at least, it did after the last treatment, and I think it will, again.

— Mark

Boceprevir

Anemia. Anemia is common during boceprevir treatment, so you are likely to need some type of treatment or intervention for anemia. There are three methods for managing anemia during treatment: reducing ribavirin dose, transfusion of red blood cells, or adding erythropoietin analogue (EPO) by weekly subcutaneous injections. In clinical trials, nearly half of the patients who had received boceprevir were treated with erythropoietin analogue (EPO). Although anemia sufficient for the institution of therapy with erythropoeitin analogue was common, discontinuation due to anemia was uncommon.

Other. While taking boceprevir, you may also experience dysgeusia, the medical term for "foul taste in the mouth." Although this symptom is annoying, it rarely leads to the discontinuation of therapy. Boceprevir is not associated with rash or anal pain.

Telaprevir

Anemia. Similar to boceprevir treatment, you are likely to experience anemia during telaprevir treatment. Yet the period of anemia attributable to telaprevir is much shorter in duration, since telaprevir is only given for 12 weeks. During the first 12 weeks of telaprevir-based triple therapy, anemia is more severe than the anemia that occurs when peginterferon/ribavirin is used without telaprevir. After the first 12 weeks, the incidence and severity of anemia due to telaprevir wears off, in which case the subsequent anemia is due to peginterferon/ribavirin. If you experience significant anemia during telaprevir treatment, your doctor may choose to manage it primarily by a dose reduction of ribavirin. This was the strategy used in the clinical trials of telaprevir. After the first 12 weeks, if anemia occurs during peginterferon/ribavirin, your doctor may choose ribavirin dose reduction, blood transfusion, or erythropoietin analogue. Rarely, you may require all three approaches to manage anemia during triple therapy.

Rash. You have about a 50 percent chance of developing skin rash during telaprevir-based treatment; the rash is mild in most cases, but occasionally can be moderate or even severe. In the clinical trials, telaprevir was discontinued in five to seven percent of patients due to moderate to severe rash. In most cases, peginterferon/ribavirin was continued so only 0.5 to 1.4 percent of patients discontinued all treatment due to rash. Rash, when it occurs, typically occurs after at least seven weeks of treatment. As shown in the ADVANCE trial, eight weeks of telaprevir may be a sufficient duration of treatment for most patients to achieve SVR. So, if you develop a rash, neither the rash or its management reduces your chance to achieve SVR.

If your rash is mild, your treating physician may recommend topical steroids (such as triamcinolone ointment), moisturizing lotions, and antihistaminics (such as hydroxyzine). If the rash involves your mouth, eyes, or internal surfaces, or if you have low blood pressure, swelling of the tissues, or asthma-like findings on a lung exam, telaprevir must be stopped immediately. A specific skin reaction, called DRESS (drug reaction with eosinophilia and systemic symptoms), is another indication to stop telaprevir. If you experience a severe rash, you may even need to be admitted to the hospital, and receive fluids and high-dose oral or intravenous steroids (Figure 5G).

FIGURE 5G: RASH DURING TELAPREVIR TREATMENT

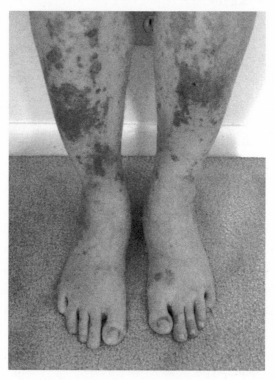

FIGURE 5G: Example of moderately severe rash during telaprevir treatment.

After the ninth week, I developed a bad skin rash all over my body. I also had extreme fatigue, but I was hopeful that treatment would cure my hepatitis C, and I kept going. The skin rash was the worst. I just got along. I couldn't work for two months—luckily, I had private disability insurance. Topical creams didn't help much, although some reduced the amount of itching.

The rash was the worst part of treatment. I am still having skin problems a couple years later. The one cream that worked the best is the

Eucerin® Calming Cream. I tried everything else, and, even now, the rash comes back if I am not using the Eucerin® cream.

— Paul

Anal Pain. Anal pain, with a burning quality, is a peculiar and very annoying side effect of telaprevir. Although annoying, anal pain rarely leads to a discontinuation of treatment. The cause is unknown, but is not due to inflammation or damage of the anus or rectum. Treatment may require topical analgesics, suppositories, lidocaine gel, stool softeners, or medications.

Try to forget about the side-effects and concentrate on the end-game. If it's going to work, it will change your life and expand your life expectancy.

— Martin

WHAT IS THE COST OF TRIPLE THERAPY?

Triple therapy is expensive. In the United States, the costs of treatment may vary between and within regions of the country. The cost figures used in the following discussion represent only crude estimates.

Telaprevir

The cost of telaprevir is approximately $4,000/week. The cost of a 12 week course would be $48,000. This is the cost just for telaprevir, and does not include costs of peginterferon, ribavirin, laboratory tests, physician fees, or clinic visits—the latter costs are approximately $3,000/month. A treatment course of 24 weeks costs approximately $66,000, and a treatment course of 48 weeks costs approximately $84,000.

Boceprevir.

The cost of boceprevir is approximately $1,200/week, and the cost of peginterferon/ribavirin is $3,000/month. The cost of 24 weeks of boceprevir would be $28,800, and the cost of 44 weeks would be $52,800. Four weeks of lead-in, followed by 24 weeks of boceprevir/

peginterferon/ribavirin, would cost $49,800. Four weeks of lead-in, followed by 44 weeks of boceprevir/peginterferon/ribavirin, would cost $88,800.

HCV GENOTYPE 1 SUBTYPES

My doctor says I have infection with HCV genotype 1b. I went to a support group, and one of the men said he had HCV genotype 1a infection. What is the difference between 1a and 1b? Do they respond differently to treatment?

— Amy

When treatment was limited to peginterferon/ribavirin without boceprevir or telaprevir, we did not appreciate consistent differences in rates of SVR between HCV genotype 1 subtypes. Now, with the advent of triple therapy, we are beginning to note some important differences.

First, in some (but not all) studies of triple therapy using a protease inhibitor in the regimen, rates of SVR are higher with HCV genotype 1b compared to HCV genotype 1a. These differences in SVR between HCV subtypes have been modest: usually only 5 percent or less.

Second (and more importantly), the risk for emergence of HCV variants that are resistant to the administered protease inhibitor is consistently lower for HCV genotype 1b. The lower risk of resistance for 1b is related to genetic differences between the 1b and 1a subtypes.

You may derive some clinical benefit if you have HCV genotype 1b infection, compared to HCV genotype 1a infection. The higher barrier to resistance of HCV genotype 1b means you might have greater chance for SVR during triple therapy. In addition, by having infection with HCV genotype 1b, compared to 1a, you are more likely to be cured by future treatment with interferon-free, ribavirin-free, dual-antiviral therapy (see chapter 6). The patient infected with HCV genotype 1a who fails to respond to current treatment may require future treatment with multi-drug regimens, such as two direct-acting antivirals with peginterferon/ribavirin (see chapter 6).

VIRAL RESISTANCE

Tell me more about viral resistance and viral variants. How do you detect the resistant viral variants? What is their importance?

—Ben

It is estimated that, in the average HCV infection, the virus replicates (creates new viruses) at a rate of approximately one trillion copies each day. During this replication process, mistakes are made in processing the genetic code of HCV, and some of these mistakes result in variant viruses that are still capable of replication to a greater or lesser extent. Generally, these variants exist in all patients, and are only uncovered by the use of drugs that inhibit the replication of the dominant and most fit virus, also called "wild-type" virus. Boceprevir and telaprevir are most active against the dominant "wild-type" HCV.

Inhibition of the wild-type virus by protease inhibitors such as boceprevir and telaprevir may allow the resistant variants to emerge as a dominant species of HCV. In the laboratory, these variants are identified by sophisticated genetic tests. In the clinic, the emergence of resistant variants of HCV is detected by rebound in HCV RNA during the course of antiviral treatment. The following is an example of emergence of resistant HCV.

Detecting Viral Resistance in the Clinic

You may be taking telaprevir/peginterferon/ribavirin, and HCV RNA is undetectable at treatment week four. Then, at treatment week eight, HCV RNA becomes detectable: HCV re-emerges despite ongoing use of triple therapy. In another example, you may experience rapid decline in HCV RNA to 500 IU/mL by treatment week four, but then, at treatment week eight, HCV RNA has rebounded 2500 IU/ml: the decline in HCV RNA ceases and begins to increase. Both of these clinical scenarios are examples of the emergence of resistant variants of HCV.

If you develop HCV resistance, it is important to immediately discontinue the protease inhibitor. If you develop resistance to boceprevir, you will be resistant to telaprevir and vice versa. Upon removal of the protease inhibitor, HCV reverts back to wild-type over the course of several months to years (slower for HCV genotype 1a). The concern regarding viral resistance is resistant viral variants may dictate your response to future courses of antiviral treatment with the next generation of drugs for the treatment of HCV. For example, if you develop resistance during either boceprevir or telaprevir, you may be resistant to re-treatment with future triple therapy using different protease inhibitors within the same class as boceprevir or telaprevir.

> *I was supposed to start boceprevir, but I had been treated with telaprevir-based triple therapy, and my HCV RNA during that treatment was immediately undetectable, and then rebounded while I was still taking telaprevir. My doctor told me that I had likely developed resistance to telaprevir, and that my HCV would also be resistant to boceprevir. He told me that I was not a good candidate for re-treatment with boceprevir because of this resistance.*

> *—Jim*

Sequential use of direct-acting antivirals, especially if used as monotherapy, could potentially favor the emergence of variants of HCV with multi-drug resistance. In contrast, use of combinations of drugs with different loci of action would reduce the risk of emergence of multi-drug resistance. Regimens, combining inhibitors of NS3/4A protease, NS5B polymerase, and NS5A, with and without peginterferon and/or ribavirin, are currently under investigation (see chapter 6).

How can you avoid or minimize the risk of viral resistance? Factors favoring the emergence of viral resistance to a protease inhibitor during triple therapy include low plasma concentrations of not only the protease inhibitor, but also low concentrations of peginterferon and possibly ribavirin. Emergence of resistant HCV is one reason that dose reduction of either boceprevir or telaprevir is not recommended. If you are intolerant of boceprevir or telaprevir, the dose of the drug must not be reduced, but rather, the drug must be discontinued. Many HCV variants resistant to boceprevir or telaprevir are sensitive to peginterferon/ribavirin. For this reason, dose reduction of peginterferon or ribavirin for the side effects of these drugs lowers their blood concentrations, and can increase the risk for the emergence of HCV variants resistant to boceprevir or telaprevir. It is critical that you be compliant with all of your triple therapy medications: peginterferon, ribavirin, and telaprevir or boceprevir.

Other clinical factors may also favor the emergence of resistant HCV variants. These include a lack of adherence to treatment, advanced liver disease, HIV, and immunosuppression.

I couldn't have done this without my wife. She is very supportive. My business partners also know about this and were very supportive. It's okay to talk about it, and that's important, because, if you are depressed and don't talk about it, you can get sicker. You are only as sick as your secrets. People are so ashamed to have this disease, as if they did something wrong.

— Ben

CONCLUDING REMARKS

Triple therapy is the new standard of care for patients infected with HCV genotype 1. Rates of SVR should approach 75 percent, and up to two-thirds of patients will only need six months of treatment. With new treatments, however, come new challenges. Side effects, such as rash and anemia, require new management strategies. Prevention of viral resistance will require that patients are carefully monitored, and that adherence to the treatment regimens be emphasized. Boceprevir and telaprevir have ushered in a new era in the treatment of HCV. If you are infected with HCV, current and future options are very promising. We may soon be entering an age when nearly every patient with chronic hepatitis C can be cured of this potentially deadly infection.

6

THE FUTURE OF HCV TREATMENT

Beyond Triple Therapy

I am still on treatment and almost halfway through the trial. I do not have hepatitis C at the present time. I hope this treatment has cured it, and I hope I will not need future treatment. The results were immediate. Before I began the QUAD Therapy clinical trial, there were over four million copies of the virus per milliliter of my blood. After the first week, that was down to only 160 copies per milliliter, and, at week two, I tested negative for hepatitis C. The virus is still undetectable in my blood—hopefully, this is it, and I am cured.

— Mark

TWENTY YEARS ago, I treated patients with HCV genotype 1 infection with interferon monotherapy, and five percent achieved SVR. Results improved to an SVR of 45 percent with peginterferon/ribavirin. Now, the new standard of care of triple therapy is expected to raise SVR up to 75 percent. What's next?

In this chapter, I look to the future, focusing on the next generation of direct-acting antivirals: new protease inhibitors, polymerase inhibitors,

NS5A inhibitors, and others. The future for treating HCV is, indeed, bright. Hopefully, the time will soon arrive when nearly every person infected with HCV will have safe, tolerable, and effective options for treatment.

The year 2011 marked the beginning of a new era in the treatment of the hepatitis C virus (HCV) with the introduction of telaprevir and boceprevir. These two drugs are inhibitors of the HCV NS3/4A protease, and are the first FDA-approved direct-acting antivirals for chronic hepatitis C. They will not be the last. Many pharmaceutical companies have targeted several HCV proteins (including the NS3/4A protease), and multiple new compounds and effective strategies are either under development or already entering later phases of testing in clinical trials.

In this chapter, I will discuss the following topics:

- Status of Clinical Investigation into Future HCV Therapies
- Next Generation Triple Therapy
    - Lambda interferon
    - Inhibitors of NS3/4A protease
    - Inhibitors of NS5B polymerase
    - Inhibitors of NS5A protein
- Interferon-Free Regimens
    - Mericitabine plus danoprevir
    - Daclatasvir plus BMS-650032
    - BI-201335 plus BI-207127 ± ribavirin
    - GS-7977 plus ribavirin
    - Genotype 1b versus 1a
- QUAD Therapy
    - Daclatasvir plus BMS-650032 plus peginterferon/ribavirin
    - Telaprevir plus VX-222 plus peginterferon/ribavirin
- Host-Acting Antivirals
    - Cyclophyllin inhibitors
    - Entry blockers
    - Micro-RNA inhibitors
- Viral Resistance
- Concluding Remarks

The ongoing developments in the treatment of chronic hepatitis C will be discussed in this chapter. Although the material in the following pages may give you a glimpse into future treatments, this is not an exhaustive review of all the possibilities. Instead, I have focused on those therapies that progressed furthest in Phase II or Phase III clinical trials. Promising drugs that are at earlier stages of development or with less clinical data may not be included in the following discussion.

WARNING: You should understand that the treatments discussed in this chapter are experimental, currently under investigation, and at various stages of testing in clinical trials. None of the treatments described in this chapter have received approval from the FDA, and, therefore, you cannot be prescribed these treatments. The only access to these treatments is through participation in clinical trials. You can check www.clinicaltrials. gov to see which trials are registered and available within your region. Also, because the treatments described in this chapter are experimental, they may be proven to be ineffective or toxic, and it is possible that only a minority of these drugs may successfully emerge for treatment of HCV in clinics.

STATUS OF CLINICAL INVESTIGATION INTO FUTURE HCV THERAPIES

I have no symptoms, my laboratory tests are normal, and my doctor says I have minimal liver disease. I want to wait and be treated with more effective drugs that have fewer side effects. I've heard there are new drugs in the pipeline. Which ones are in clinical trials and show potential promise for emerging or future treatments?

— *Robert*

Currently, the field of hepatology is hyper-focused on the treatment of hepatitis C. Hepatitis C was listed as the main topic of 541 abstracts at the 2011 meeting of the American Association for the Study of Liver Diseases, representing 24 percent of the entire meeting. Three hundred and nine abstracts were focused on clinical trials or treatment of chronic hepatitis C, representing 13 percent of the meeting. In addition, scanning websites revealed a plethora of activity, including 285 registrations on clinicaltrials.gov. At hcvdrugs.com, there were listings for eight trials of combination treatments, 96 trials of single direct–acting antivirals, and 37 trials of immune modulators. At hcvadvocate.com, there were listings for 10 Phase I trials, 19 Phase II trials, and four Phase III trials. Another outstanding website with current information on treatments for HCV is www.natap.org. There are many additional websites devoted to hepatitis C and evolving treatments. I recommend that you take efforts to stay informed by visiting these sites periodically. New, more tolerable, and more potent drug therapies for chronic hepatitis C and HCV will undoubtedly be a future reality[88] (Figure 6A).

FIGURE 6A: EMERGING TREATMENTS
(ABSTRACTS AT AASLD 2011)

	↑eRVR	↑SVR	↓SEs	↓Pills	↓Freq	NoIFN
TT Regimens with PR						
TMC-435	√	±	√	√	qd	-
BI -201335	√	±	√	√	qd	-
BMS-790052	√	+	√	√	qd	-
PSI-7977 G1	√	++	√	√	qd	-
PSI-7977 G2/3	√	++	√	√	qd	√
Danoprevir	√	++	?	√	bid	-
Vaniprevir	?	+	?	√	bid	-
Narlaprevir/rtv	√	++	√	√	qd	-
QUAD Regimens						
BMS (PR+NS5A-I+PI)	√	+++	±	√	DAAs qd	-
VX (PR+PI+NNI)	√	+++	±	-	-	-
IFN-Free Regimens						
BMS (NS5A-I+PI) G1 a/b	±	±	√	√	qd	√
BMS (NS5A-I+PI) G1b	√	+++	?	√	qd	√
BI (PI+NNI+RBV)	√	?	√	√	qd	√
PSI (NI+RBV) G2/3	√	+++	√	√	qd	√
Alisporivir ± RBV G2/3	-	?	√	±	qd	√

FIGURE 6A: This table lists some, but not all, of the emerging treatment options for chronic hepatitis C. A checkmark in a given column indicates enhancement of eRVR and SVR, or reduction in side effects, number of pills, frequency of dosing of the direct acting antiviral, and the possibility of IFN-free treatment. The regimens listed were presented in part at the last meeting of the American Association for the Study of Liver Diseases (AASLD 2011).

My advice to anyone who is considering a trial is simple: just keep going. The more attention you give to how badly you feel, the worse it becomes. Just maintain your daily routine throughout the trial, and try to keep on track with your life and commitments. Strictly follow the protocol and live your life.

— Barb

The first week, the virus was cleared. I won't know whether I am still infected until I complete this round of therapy, though. If I test clear six months after I complete the therapy (and I hope I do), I will be considered cured. But, for now, I'm still in the thick of it. I'll know for sure in about a year. If I still have hepatitis C, I would try another trial. There are so many clinical trials going on; there are about 75 throughout the country. It's a very dynamic time for hepatitis C research. Sooner or later, someone will hit the Holy Grail of hepatitis C treatment. I may very well be in the trial that is the cure.

— *Frank*

Stick it out. I put needles in my arm for many years, and I was strung out. I'm drug-free for over 27 years, and that was a big accomplishment. But doing this clinical trial is the greatest accomplishment in my life. You don't hear the word "cure" used for anything. Now, it's being used as "hepatitis C cure." So, the chance that I will be cured of this is worth any of the side effects. Plus, I have come to appreciate the staff who are treating me—they are phenomenal. I have to keep going.

— *Butch*

NEXT GENERATION TRIPLE THERAPY

Some of the emerging regimens contain the backbone of peginterferon and ribavirin, typically when the regimen includes a single direct-acting antiviral. The single direct-acting antiviral could be a NS3/4A protease inhibitor, NS5B polymerase inhibitor, or NS5A inhibitor. These regimens are the next generation of triple therapy.

Lambda Interferon

If triple therapy remains the standard of care for the foreseeable future, then new options for the peginterferon/ribavirin backbone may be developed. The current interferons that are FDA-approved for treatment of chronic hepatitis C are alfa interferons, including peginterferon alfa-2a, peginterferon alfa-2b, consensus interferon, interferon alfa-2a, and interferon alfa-2b. Lambda interferon is a relatively new type of interferon that has also shown promise in the treatment of chronic hepatitis C[89, 90]. A pegylated form of lambda interferon (PEGIFN-lambda) is completing Phase II clinical trials, and likely will soon move to Phase III testing.

PEGIFN-lambda may have greater antiviral potency than the alfa peginterferons and, perhaps more importantly, fewer side effects. PEGIFN-lambda inhibits the bone marrow less than the alfa interferons. Why is that good? Your bone marrow produces all of your blood cells: red blood cells, white blood cells, and platelets. Compared to alfa-interferons, patients taking lambda interferon have less anemia (lowering of red blood cells), and maintain higher levels of white blood cells (the cells that fight infection) and platelets (the cells that aid clotting). The main clinical benefits of these effects could include a reduced need for ribavirin dose reduction, less transfusion of red blood cells, and decreased use of treatments to raise red blood cells (erythropoietin analogues) or white blood cells (granulocyte-colony stimulating factors). PEGIFN-lambda might be a better tolerated interferon for use with emerging triple therapy regimens.

Inhibitors of NS3/4A Protease

As you learned from reading chapters 4 and 5 of this book, the first two direct-acting antivirals to be FDA-approved for treating hepatitis C, telaprevir and boceprevir, are NS3/4A protease inhibitors. Clearly, telaprevir and boceprevir enhance the treatment of chronic hepatitis C. Yet both require interferon/ribavirin, are active mainly against HCV genotype 1, and side effects are an issue. For these reasons, there remains great interest in the development of additional protease inhibitors with greater potency, fewer side effects, and activity against all HCV genotypes.

TMC-435. TMC-435 is a new protease inhibitor that has just begun Phase III clinical trials[91, 92, 93]. In Phase II trials, up to 86 percent of patients treated with TMC-435-based triple therapy achieved eRVR, and were thus eligible for early discontinuation of treatment at 24 weeks. Also, the maximum reported SVR was 86 percent, and TMC-435 was not associated with rash or the lowering of white blood cells, red blood cells, or platelets. During treatment, some patients did experience an increase in bilirubin without evidence of liver damage. The increase in bilirubin was stable during treatment, and resolved itself after the discontinuation of TMC-435. The Phase II studies suggest that triple therapy with TMC-435 appears to be highly effective and well-tolerated. Phase III trials with TMC-435 are ongoing.

BI-201335. BI-201335 is another new protease inhibitor that has just begun Phase III clinical trials[94, 95]. In the Phase II trials, up to 87 percent of patients treated with BI-201335-based triple therapy achieved eRVR, and were thus eligible for early discontinuation of treatment at 24 weeks. The maximum reported SVR was 83 percent, and BI-201335 was not associated with any additional or new adverse effects. As with TMC-435, transient elevations in bilirubin were reported, and, in the Phase II trials, triple therapy with BI-201335 also appeared to be highly effective and well-tolerated. Phase III trials with BI-201335 are ongoing.

Danoprevir (RG-7227). Danoprevir is also highly effective[96, 97]. In the Phase II trial, ATLAS, eRVR was 79 percent, and SVR was 85 percent for danoprevir-based (600 milligrams twice daily) triple therapy. In the ATLAS trial, a high dose arm of 900 milligrams twice daily was associated with alanine aminotransferase (ALT) elevations, and this arm was closed prematurely. To address the ALT elevation and also enhance potency, danoprevir is now being studied with ritonavir (RTV) in clinical trials. The Phase II results of triple therapy using danoprevir/RTV are encouraging (DAUPHINE trial, SVR 12 up to 93 percent [EASL 2012]).

Narlaprevir/Ritonavir (RTV)[98]. In a recent Phase II trial, triple therapy with narlaprevir/RTV yielded a maximum SVR of 85 percent. Ritonavir boosted the potency of narlaprevir by altering its metabolism in the body, allowing once daily dosing, and it also reduced side effects. The status of development of narlaprevir is unclear.

Many other protease inhibitors are proceeding down the path of clinical development. These include vaniprevir, BMS-650032, GS-9256,

ACH-1625, IDX-320, VX-985, and ABT-450. Many of these compounds appear very promising as potent and well-tolerated inhibitors of the HCV NS3/4A protease.

Inhibitors of NS5B Polymerase

Polymerase inhibitors target the NS5B RNA-dependent RNA polymerase of HCV, an enzyme critical for viral replication. There are two types of polymerase inhibitors: nucleoside or non-nucleoside. Nucleoside inhibitors target the active site of NS5B in a competitive manner, have broad spectrum activity, and lead to RNA chain termination. Non-nucleoside inhibitors bind at a site distant to the catalytic center of the polymerase. An increased genetic barrier to resistance is reported for the nucleoside inhibitors, while the non-nucleoside inhibitors have had significant issues with resistance and suboptimal viral suppression.

Mericitabine (RG-7128). Mericitabine is a cytidine nucleoside analog[99, 100]. In Phase I trials of HCV genotype 1 non-responders, 14 days of treatment with mericitabine produced a $2.7\log_{10}$ IU/mL decline in viral load at a dose of 1,500 milligrams twice daily. No serious adverse effects were reported in the treatment group. Subsequent trials of mericitabine in combination with peginterferon/ribavirin demonstrated a $5\log_{10}$ IU/mL decline in HCV RNA by week four of treatment.

Results from the JUMP-C trial indicated an SVR at week 12 of 76 percent for response-guided therapy with mericitibine-based triple therapy. Importantly, there was no evidence of the emergence of breakthrough related to viral resistance. Mericitibine is undergoing further investigation in combination with danoprevir.

> *The treatment of my hepatitis C with peginterferon, ribavirin, and the new drug (mericitabine) is best described as the worst case of flu I've ever had—but now I'm over it, and, lucky for me, no hepatitis C.*
>
> — *Terry*

GS-7977. GS-7977 is a potent nucleoside (pyrimidine) NS5B polymerase inhibitor that has generated intense interest as a potential breakthrough in HCV treatment[93, 100, 101, 102]. In a Phase II study, PROTON, GS-7977-based triple therapy was evaluated in 121 treatment-naïve patients with HCV genotype 1 infection (Figure 6B). Stages of fibrosis ranged from F0 to F2 (mild fibrosis), and there were only a few black patients. This regimen was quite potent: 98 percent of patients at week four of treatment had undetectable HCV RNA. The SVR at week 12 reported at AASLD 2011 was 91 percent. These encouraging results have catapulted GS-7977 into the forefront of emerging HCV therapies—the pharmaceutical company, Gilead Sciences, purchased the maker of GS-7977, Pharmasset, for $11 billion. GS-7977-based triple therapy is beginning Phase III trials.

NOTE: When Gilead purchased Pharmasset, PSI-7977 was changed to GS-7977.

FIGURE 6B: RESULTS FROM THE PROTON STUDY OF GS-7977 TREATMENT-NAIVE PATIENTS WITH HCV GENOTYPE I

%

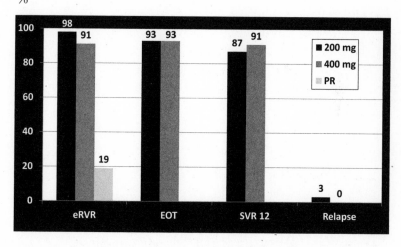

No new safety events. There were 3 viral breakthroughs and 1 relapse in the 200mg arm. All 4 were CT by IL28b polymorphism.

FIGURE 6B: The results of the PROTON study are shown (as presented at AASLD 2011). SVR 12 was highly favorable (91 percent) with a regimen of GS-7977/peginterferon/ribavirin. GS-7977 is a nucleoside NS5B polymerase inhibitor.

An advantage of HCV polymerase inhibitors is they may be active against non-1 HCV genotypes. Mericitabine, GS-7977, PSI-938, and other NS5B polymerase inhibitors have activity against non-1 HCV genotypes.

Several additional polymerase inhibitors are at various stages of clinical investigation. These include VX-222, GS-9190, PSI-7792, BI-207127, IDX-375, IDX-184, ALS-2200, ALS-2158, MK-0608, TMC-649128, PF-868554, ANA-598, VCH-759, ABT-837093, ABT-072, ABT-333, INX-189, and GSK-625433. Many of these compounds appear very promising as potent and well-tolerated inhibitors of the HCV NS5B polymerase.

Inhibitors of NS5A Protein

Daclatasvir (BMS-790052). NS5A is an HCV protein with no known enzymatic function, but is a co-factor in HCV replication[103, 104, 105]. The drug daclatasvir (BMS-790052) has demonstrated potent inhibition of NS5A and HCV replication. In a placebo-controlled trial of 48 treatment-naïve patients with HCV genotype 1, SVR at week 12 was 92 percent (11 out of 12 patients) with 10 milligrams per day for 48 weeks, and 83 percent (10 out of 12 patients) with 60 milligrams per day for 48 weeks of daclatasvir. Side effects and adverse events were similar between treatment and control arms. Daclatasvir is being studied in a triple therapy regimen in ongoing Phase III trials.

Other NS5A inhibitors are in early phases of clinical trials. These include ACH-2928, PPI-461, AZD-7295, and others. Once again, many appear promising as components of triple therapy or other combination treatments.

INTERFERON-FREE REGIMENS

With the explosion of new direct-acting antivirals for HCV, the dream of interferon-free treatment is edging closer to clinical reality. As you know, the side effects of interferon and the burden of injections dominate management issues for patients and providers. Elimination of interferon could greatly simplify the treatment regimen, and improve patient adherence and compliance. Several interferon-free protocols are currently under clinical investigation.

I'm glad I was able to get into a trial that was interferon-free. Interferon is brutal; I had numerous side effects during my last treatment with peginterferon and ribavirin. Now I understand what women experience when they have bad PMS. The mood swings come so suddenly, and your reactions are so quick and uncontrollable.

I've had very dry skin, anxiety, extreme fatigue, and depression. I coped with the help of my family and the staff at the clinic. I had trouble sleeping, too, so I was given 50 milligrams of Trazadone to help with sleep.

— *Michael*

Mericitabine Plus Danoprevir

INFORM was the first clinical trial to investigate the efficacy of the combination of a protease inhibitor with a polymerase inhibitor.[99] This Phase I double-blinded ascending dose trial investigated the combination of 14 days of the polymerase inhibitor, mericitabine, with the protease inhibitor, danoprevir. Some patients were treatment-naïve, and others had previous therapy with interferon-based regimens. Significant viral load decline was noted over 14 days, with a median reduction in viral levels of 4.8 to 5.2 $\log_{10}$ IU/mL. Sixty-three percent of treatment-naïve and 25 percent of prior null responders receiving dual therapy were HCV RNA negative at 14 days. Further studies are underway to modify and better define this treatment regimen. This combination, with and without peginterferon or ribavirin, is currently under investigation in the MATTERHORN trial.

Daclatasvir Plus BMS-650032

This combination of inhibitors of NS5A protein and NS3/4A protease was studied in 11 null responders to prior treatment with peginterferon/ribavirin who were infected with HCV genotype 1[106]. All 11 patients demonstrated a brisk decline in HCV RNA, and four achieved

SVR despite only 24 weeks of treatment. The only breakthroughs were patients with HCV subtype 1a. Neither of the two patients with HCV subtype 1b experienced breakthrough.

This combination, given for twenty-four weeks, was also used in a study of ten Japanese null responders, all of whom were infected with HCV subtype 1b. The SVR was 100 percent[104]. Interferon-free, ribavirin-free dual DAA therapy may become a reality for patients infected with HCV genotype 1b (Figure 6C).

FIGURE 6C: DUAL INHIBITION OF NS5A PROTEIN AND NS3/4A PROTEASE

10 JAPANESE NULL RESPONDERS WITH HCV GENOTYPE 1B

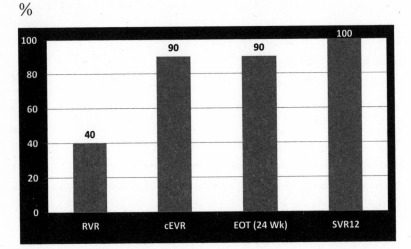

Baseline RAVs to BMS-790052 and BMS-650032 did not affect response to treatment. 1 patient who stopped at week 2, and the 9 who took 24 weeks achieved SVR12.

FIGURE 6C: A pilot study of interferon-free, ribavirin-free treatment using DUAL inhibition of NS5A protein and NS3/4A protease was highly effective in 10 Japanese patients infected with HCV genotype 1b who had a prior null response to peginterferon/ribavirin.

Although daclatasvir/BMS-650032 may be very effective against the subtype 1b of HCV genotype 1, it is less effective against subtype 1a. For subtype 1a, daclatasvir/BMS-650032 will likely need to be combined with other drugs (such as peginterferon, ribavirin, or other direct-acting antivirals) to provide additional potency and broader activity.

BI-201335 Plus BI-207127 ± Ribavirin

Potential efficacy of this regimen was first suggested from the results of the SOUND-C1 trial[94]. SOUND-C2 is an ongoing Phase II study of three interferon-free regimens: two with ribavirin and one without. The patients were infected with HCV genotype 1 and were treatment-naïve. All arms received a single daily dose of BI-201335. In the ribavirin-free arm, BI-207127 was given three times daily. In one ribavirin-containing arm, BI-207127 was also given three times daily, and, in the remaining ribavirin-containing arm, it was given twice daily. Virologic responses have been higher in the two arms containing ribavirin, suggesting that ribavirin may be required in interferon-free treatment regimens. On-treatment virologic responses have been brisk: up to 88 percent had cleared HCV RNA by week four of treatment and up to 82 percent achieved SVR 12 (EASL 2012).

GS-7977 Plus Ribavirin

This 12-week interferon-free dual regimen was used in 10 treatment-naïve patients with HCV genotype 2/3 infection[102]. The regimen was well-tolerated with few side effects, and 100 percent of the patients achieved SVR, despite the very short course of only 12 weeks of treatment.

After these results were known, a small exploratory study of GS-7977 monotherapy (no ribavirin or interferon) for genotype 2/3 patients was undertaken. On-treatment responses were brisk, but some patients broke through or relapsed. Thus, it appears that ribavirin may be required for optimal virologic responses with GS-7977 when used in interferon-free protocols.

ABT-450/r Plus ABT-333 Plus Ribavirin

This 12-week interferon-free triple regimen was used in a pilot study of 33 treatment-naïve patients and 17 prior nonresponders to peginterferon/ribavirin—all with HCV genotype 1 infection. The regimen was well-tolerated with few side effects. Up to 95 percent of the treatment-naïve patients and 47 percent of the treatment-experienced patients achieved SVR12—with only 12 weeks of treatment and no interferon (EASL 2012)! Additional studies with this combination and other drugs are ongoing.

A number of interferon-free regimens, with and without ribavirin, are currently under study. Some of the combinations of direct-acting antivirals include telaprevir with VX-222, GS-9190 with GS-9256, IDX-184 with IDX-320, BMS-790052 with BMS-650032, BI-201335 with BI-207127, mericitibine with danoprevir, and GS-7977 with PSI-938. Many of these combinations appear promising as interferon-free treatments.

Genotype 1b Versus 1a

HCV genotype 1b, compared to 1a, may be particularly responsive or susceptible to interferon-free treatment. There is something very different about HCV genotypes 1a and 1b: the barrier for emergence of viral variants resistant to the protease inhibitors is higher for HCV genotype 1b. This means, during treatment of a patient infected with HCV genotype 1a, resistant viral variants may emerge that compromise virologic response. This translates to a lower chance for cure with interferon-free treatment regimens in patients infected with HCV genotype 1a. Do not be alarmed if you have HCV genotype 1a infection, as the rates of SVR are excellent with many of the new treatments. Nonetheless, maximizing your chances to achieve SVR if you are infected with HCV genotype 1a may require multi-drug regimens and peginterferon.

QUAD THERAPY

QUAD therapy implies the use of two direct-acting antivirals with peginterferon/ribavirin. The early experience with QUAD therapy in a very small number of patients has been promising. QUAD therapy dramatically enhances SVR and also blocks the emergence of resistant viral variants.

Daclatasvir Plus BMS-650032 Plus Peginterferon/Ribavirin

This combination of inhibitors of NS5A and NS3/4A protease plus peginterferon/ribavirin was studied in 10 null responders to prior treatment with peginterferon/ribavirin who were infected with HCV genotype 1, mostly subtype 1a (Figure 6D). Nine of the 10 patients achieved SVR despite only 24 weeks of treatment. Additional studies of this QUAD regimen are underway.

FIGURE 6D: QUAD THERAPY OF NULL RESPONDERS (N=10)
WITH HCV GENOTYPE I
NS5A AND NS3/4A INHIBITORS + PR FOR 24 WEEKS

% HCV RNA <10 IU/ML

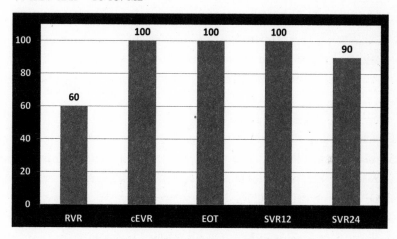

Lok A, et al. N Engl J Med 2012;366:216-224.

FIGURE 6D: These preliminary results in 10 patients suggest that QUAD treatment may be effective in re-treatment of HCVgenotype 1a and 1b null responders. QUAD included inhibitors of NS5A protein and NS3/4A protease with peginterferon/ribavirin.

Telaprevir Plus VX-222 Plus Peginterferon/Ribavirin

This combination of NS3/4A protease inhibitor, NS5B non-nucleoside polymerase inhibitor, and peginterferon/ribavirin was tested in 59 treatment-naïve patients infected with HCV genotype 1. There was a very interesting twist to this study: the patients who had a very rapid virologic response (vRVR), defined as undetectable HCV RNA at weeks two through eight stopped treatment at week 12. Fifty percent of the patients achieved vRVR and stopped all treatment at week 12. Ninety-three percent of those patients then went on to achieve SVR. Those not achieving vRVR were given an additional 12 weeks of peginterferon/ribavirin. The overall rate of SVR for all patients on this QUAD regimen was 90 percent.

> *The virus is gone, and has not been detected. I will get blood work every two weeks. As of today, I am not infected. As of today, I am cured. I never had a treatment clear the virus before . . . not even close. So, I feel as though it's cured. We'll know for sure after six months, but, as of today, I am not infected. If, in six months, I still have the virus, I would treat, again. I have complete faith that, ultimately, I will be cured of this infection—if not now, in the future.*
>
> — *Gary*

Additional QUAD regimens are currently under study. QUAD therapy may push the limits of SVR to near 100 percent, and will likely cover the broad range of genotypes and subtypes. The high potency of QUAD therapy reduces the need for baseline predictors of response (such as IL28B polymorphism), prevents the emergence of resistant viral variants, and allows further shortening of the duration of the antiviral therapy.

HOST-ACTING ANTIVIRALS

Interferon was actually the first host-acting antiviral to be used clinically in the treatment of HCV. Interferons exert their antiviral effects via interaction with specific receptors on your cells, which then triggers a number of reactions aimed at clearing HCV. Interferons are not directly antiviral, since they do not bind to HCV or directly attack the replication of HCV. Instead, interferons activate a number of antiviral genes within your cells, which then inhibit various pathways necessary for viral replication. A number of additional host targets beyond interferon have now been identified that can inhibit HCV or aid in its clearance.

Cyclophyllin Inhibitors

Cyclophyllin is a common cellular protein that plays an important role in facilitating the replication of HCV. Cyclophyllin interacts with both NS5B polymerase and NS5A protein to enhance viral replication. Inhibitors of cyclophyllin, such as alisporivir, SCY-635, and EP-Cyp546, block the cyclophyllin-mediated HCV replication. The most extensive clinical experience is with the cyclophyllin inhibitor, alisporivir[107, 108, 109].

Entry Blockers

A number of compounds have been developed that inhibit the uptake of HCV by liver cells (hepatocytes). Although clinical development is at an early stage, this strategy could be particularly useful at or near the time of transplantation to prevent the infection of the allograft (donor liver from an unrelated person).

Micro-RNA Inhibitors

Micro-RNA inhibitors, particularly miR-122, stabilize HCV replication. An anti-sense oligonucleotide inhibitor (an RNA that binds to other RNA) of miR-122, miravirsen, was given intravenously weekly for four weeks to patients with HCV genotype 1 infection. HCV RNA declined by nearly $2\log_{10}$ IU/mL. Additional studies are planned.

A number of other host factors have been targeted for their potential antiviral effects. These include the innate immune system and vaccination strategies to enhance immune mechanisms for the recognition and clearance of HCV.

VIRAL RESISTANCE

HCV replicates at a rate of approximately one trillion copies of virus each day. During this replication process, mistakes in the transcription of the genetic code of HCV are made, and some of these mistakes result in virus that is still capable of replication, but varies from the native or "wild-type" HCV. Generally, these variants exist in all patients, and are only uncovered by the use of drugs that primarily inhibit replication of the wild-type virus. Inhibition of the wild-type virus allows the variants to emerge as a dominant species of HCV. In the laboratory, these variants are identified by sophisticated genetic sequencing. In the clinic, the emergence of resistant viral variants is detected by a rebound in HCV RNA during the course of antiviral treatment. A typical example of this would be a patient taking telaprevir/peginterferon/ribavirin, whose HCV RNA was negative at week four of treatment, and who experiences a positive HCV RNA at week eight of treatment. In another example, a patient experiences rapid decline in HCV RNA to 500 IU/mL by week four, but then has a rebound in HCV RNA to 2500 IU/ml at week eight. Both of these cases are examples of breakthrough due to the emergence of resistant viral variants.

> *I was feeling fine, with no serious side effects. During week four of treatment, I felt great, my blood tests were normal, and HCV RNA was no longer detectable—but at week eight, I received a call from my nurse to stop the medications because the virus had broken through: the HCV RNA, which was undetectable, was now 1500 IU/mL. By immediately stopping the drugs, the doctors were trying to reduce the chances that I would remain resistant to the telaprevir. In fact, over the last nine months, the viral variants of HCV that were resistant to telaprevir are no longer detectable. I have the same HCV in my blood now that I had prior to treatment.*
>
> — *Carol*

If resistance is recognized, and the protease inhibitor is discontinued, the HCV RNA reverts back to wild-type HCV RNA over the course of several months or even years (slower for HCV genotype 1a compared to 1b). The concern regarding viral resistance is resistance may dictate response to future courses of direct-acting antiviral treatment. Selection of viral variants resistant to the first-generation protease inhibitors may create new strains of HCV with broad resistance profiles. Sequential use of monotherapy protocols would favor this phenomenon, while use of combination, multi-drug regimens would tend to prevent this.

Variants of HCV resistant to the administered protease inhibitor may emerge during triple therapy. Risk factors favoring the emergence of viral resistance include low plasma concentrations of the protease inhibitor, peginterferon (and possibly ribavirin), a lack of adherence to treatment regimen, and other factors that may compromise virologic response (such as advanced liver disease, HIV, or immunosuppression). If side effects, such as those mentioned above, cause a decreased adherence to a treatment regimen, the development of resistance could be substantial. Considerations in the development of drug resistant HCV variants include an inability to obtain complete viral suppression, drug metabolism and clearance, and poor adherence to a specified triple therapy regimen resulting in lower serum levels. Prolonged monotherapy with a direct-acting agent may also result in a progressive accumulation of mutations, given the virus's high replication rate and the poor fidelity of its change to replication.

As a patient undergoing treatment, you have a role to play in preventing viral resistance. Take the direct-acting antiviral drugs and any other administered antivirals, such as interferon or ribavirin, only as prescribed. Never alter dose or dosing frequency of direct-acting antivirals: if you are not tolerating these drugs, they must be discontinued, not dose-reduced. In addition, adhere to the recommendations of your care providers regarding the dosing of interferon and ribavirin.

CONCLUDING REMARKS

Many options for the treatment of HCV are emerging. These include new NS3/4A protease inhibitors, NS5B polymerase inhibitors, NS5A inhibitors, and host-acting antivirals. These drugs and emerging combinations may further improve treatment options and enhance the outcome for patients with chronic hepatitis C. New triple therapy regimens, interferon-free treatment, QUAD therapy, and other combinations are extremely potent and seemingly well tolerated. Within the next five years, there may be treatment options that can eradicate HCV in nearly every patient.

In addition to the cited references, much of the data quoted in this chapter was extracted from abstracts and talks presented at the meeting of the European Association for the Study of the Liver in April, 2011, and the meeting of the American Association for the Study of Liver Diseases in November, 2011. These abstracts and most of the data can be found in:

1. Abstract Book from The International Liver Congress 2011. 46th annual meeting of the European Association for the Study of the Liver. *Journal of Hepatology* 2011; 54: Supplement 1.
2. Abstract Book from The Liver Meeting. 62nd Annual Meeting of the American Association for the Study of Liver Diseases. *Hepatology* 2011; October Issue.

7

RE-TREATMENT AFTER PRIOR TREATMENT WITH DIRECT-ACTING ANTIVIRALS
What Might Be the Future Options?

I took triple therapy; I received peginterferon, ribavirin, and telaprevir. With triple therapy, I cleared the hepatitis C from my blood pretty quickly, and was clear for nearly six months. Because I cleared so fast, I had eRVR, and I was able to stop my treatment after only six months. Boy, did I feel great—no hepatitis C after only six months of treatment. Then disaster struck. My first follow-up lab test came back positive for HCV RNA: only 1,100 IU/mL, but still positive. I was sure this couldn't be; there must have been some mistake; perhaps the lab accidentally switched samples? So, the test was repeated, but alas, once again, positive HCV RNA, but, now, it had climbed to 550,000 IU/mL. That wasn't too different from my baseline before I received the triple therapy. Now, I am considering future treatment options. Although I didn't clear hepatitis C, I gave my liver a rest, and feel that there will be many more options. I will get rid of hepatitis C someday. I hope to participate in another clinical trial or treatment regimen in the future.

— Sam

IN THIS chapter, I will address an important emerging issue: how to treat hepatitis C in patients who have already had a course of treatment that included one or more direct-acting antiviral drugs. Because telaprevir and boceprevir are now FDA-approved, the most common clinical situation would be a patient who has been treated with triple therapy using either telaprevir or boceprevir, and, despite this treatment, remains infected with HCV. In addition, a much smaller number of patients have now been exposed to combinations of direct-acting antivirals via clinical trials, and remain infected with HCV. At the time of this writing, there have not been any published or presented clinical data or trials related to this issue. I offer my own personal suggestions on how to evaluate, approach, and manage the patients who remain infected with HCV, despite prior treatment with direct-acting antivirals.

In this chapter, I will discuss the following topics:

- Definitions of Failure of Triple Therapy
  - Failure due to poor compliance, intolerability, or adverse events
  - Failure due to viral resistance
- Potential Options for Re-Treatment
  - Lambda interferon
  - Triple therapy using more potent protease inhibitors
  - Triple therapy using direct-acting antivirals other than protease inhibitors
  - HCV genotype 1a versus 1b
  - QUAD therapy
  - Interferon-free treatment options
- Concluding Remarks

Of the patients that have been treated with telaprevir or boceprevir-based triple therapy and remained infected with HCV, nearly all cases will be infected with HCV genotype 1. The likelihood of treatment failure during triple therapy is related to poor virologic response to peginterferon/ribavirin, an intolerability of the treatment regimen, and viral resistance to the administered protease inhibitor or other direct-acting antiviral (DAA).

Patient Category According to PEG/RBV Exposure	Percentage of Patients Still Infected with HCV Despite Triple Therapy
Naïve	25 to 35%
Relapse	10 to 25%
Partial Responder	45 to 55%
Null Responder	60 to 70%

Re-treatment after triple therapy or therapy with any direct-acting antiviral drug promises to be an increasingly important emerging issue in HCV therapy. In this chapter, I will cover some key issues regarding re-treatment of patients who remain infected with HCV despite a prior course that included a direct-acting antiviral.

WARNING: You should understand that there have not yet been any clinical trials that have addressed the issue of re-treatment of patients who remain infected after a prior course of treatment that included one or more direct-acting antiviral drugs. I have already been confronted by patients with this issue, and have decided to provide in this chapter a framework to understand the issues regarding re-treatment and which re-treatment regimens might provide the best chance for SVR. Optimum regimens for re-treatment will require investigation via properly controlled clinical trials. None of the regimens described in this chapter have been investigated or have received approval from the FDA, and, therefore, you cannot be prescribed these treatments.

DEFINITIONS OF FAILURE OF TRIPLE THERAPY

I took telaprevir, peginterferon, and ribavirin. Treatment was tough. By week six, I was extremely fatigued, and my red blood cells had bottomed out. The ribavirin was discontinued, and the doctor had to give me two blood transfusions. Even though I was beating hepatitis C, and the HCV RNA was undetectable in my blood tests, I couldn't take it any longer. I had had enough, and stopped treatment early—and, as expected, the hepatitis C returned. Now what? Do I have any other options for treatment?

— Jill

Failure Due to Poor Compliance, Intolerability, or Adverse Events

Poor Compliance. The triple therapy regimen is complicated. It includes weekly subcutaneous injections of peginterferon up to a total of 48 injections, as many as three ribavirin pills twice daily, and two pills of telaprevir or four pills of boceprevir three times daily. When taking triple therapy, you must stay on schedule, keep track of all the medications, dose properly with the correct medication, and take each of the drugs for the correct amount of time. There is plenty of room for error.

Your doctor will need to assess your compliance with your prior course of triple therapy when evaluating you for re-treatment. It is important that you provide your doctor with accurate information: be honest about the difficulties that you have had in staying on track during triple therapy. Your physician will likely ask you questions such as:

- Did you miss doses during your prior course of triple therapy?
    Of the peginterferon?
    Of the ribavirin?
    Of the telaprevir or boceprevir?
- How often did you miss doses?
- Did you take the drugs for the correct period of time?

Why do you need to answer these questions? In designing your next level of treatment, your doctor will need to know whether one or more of the drugs has been particularly difficult for you. For example, some patients are uncomfortable with the prospect of giving themselves or another person an injection. If you simply could not handle the injections, then a re-treatment regimen involving injections would not be a good choice for you. As another example, you may have been working, and found it difficult to remember to take a particular dose of either telaprevir or boceprevir, or perhaps you could not tolerate the thought of having another fatty meal with each dose. In either case, re-treatment using a direct-acting antiviral requiring three-times-daily dosing or frequent fatty meals would not be best for you. In some cases, patients lose track of ribavirin dosing. Some patients think that, because they are taking the telaprevir or boceprevir pills, they might be able to stop taking the ribavirin. As we stated in earlier chapters, that simply does not work. To be maximally effective, you must take all three drugs using their correct dosages for the proper period of time. If the complexity of the number of drugs and dosing intervals has simply been too much for you, let your provider know.

Another difficulty with adhering to triple therapy is staying on your medications for the correct period of time. The treatment schedules for triple therapy are different for telaprevir versus boceprevir, but both are complicated and require an understanding of eRVR (extended rapid virologic response). You might have been confused by the terms used by your providers—perhaps you thought you could stop treatment early due to your virologic response when, in fact, you should have continued. Or, for some other reason, you simply decided to quit. In any case, let your provider know the exact reasons for your inability to comply with the prior triple therapy regimen. After all, both you and your provider want you to be cured of hepatitis C. Designing the best re-treatment for you will require your provider to examine multiple factors, including any problems that you have had in complying with prior triple therapy.

Intolerability. Every drug in the triple therapy regimen can be associated with side effects, but your doctor will want to know which side effects of treatment have been most disconcerting and resulted in discontinuing therapy. Intolerability is a fairly common cause of a premature discontinuation of treatment.

You may have experienced severe flu-like symptoms, marked mood alteration, or extreme fatigue, and stopped due to these side effects. If these symptoms were the problem, then your decision to stop treatment was likely due to side effects from peginterferon. The peginterferons currently approved by the FDA for treatment of HCV are alfa interferons. A new interferon, lambda interferon, is also pegylated, proceeding through Phase II and III clinical trials, and seems to have fewer side effects than the alfa interferons. So, your re-treatment regimen might need to substitute lambda peginterferon for alfa peginterferon or be free of any of the peginterferons altogether.

Anemia. Anemia (low counts of red blood cells) is a very common issue, and all of the drugs in triple therapy contribute to anemia. Ribavirin causes the breakdown of circulating red blood cells (hemolysis), and peginterferon, boceprevir, and telaprevir block the ability of the bone marrow to produce enough red blood cells to build up the circulating mass of red blood cells. Over the many years that I have treated patients with chronic hepatitis C, I have witnessed varying ranges of the severity of anemia occurring with various treatments. Anemia is rare when peginterferon is used alone, moderate with the combination of peginterferon and ribavirin, and most severe with triple therapy (either telaprevir or boceprevir-based). If severe anemia was a key factor leading to the discontinuation of your prior course of triple therapy, then your re-treatment regimen will need to include direct-acting antivirals with little to no effect on your bone marrow, or be peginterferon-free, ribavirin-free, or both peginterferon and ribavirin-free.

Rash. Rash is rarely due to peginterferon, is more common with ribavirin, not associated with boceprevir, but very common with telaprevir. Severe rash is nearly exclusively due to telaprevir, and patients experiencing severe rash during telaprevir-based triple therapy should avoid telaprevir in any re-treatment regimen.

Anal pain. Although anal pain is a common aggravating symptom of telaprevir, it rarely leads to discontinuation. The same may be stated for the dysgeusia (foul taste in mouth) of boceprevir. Symptoms of anal pain or dysgeusia during a prior course of telaprevir or boceprevir-based triple therapy would not necessarily exclude telapreir, boceprevir, or other DAAs with these side effects from inclusion in re-treatment regimens.

NOTE: There are no absolute guidelines. Your doctor will need to weigh complex issues when he designs the optimal re-treatment regimen for you, as these decisions likely will be highly individualized. What works for another patient may not be ideal for you. In designing re-treatment, your doctor may decide that the benefit of using peginterferon, ribavirin, or a specific direct-acting antiviral on improving your chance for SVR and cure outweighs the risks related to anemia or other side effects that you may have experienced during prior triple therapy. Your doctor essentially accepts the fact that he will need to manage anemia or other side effects during your re-treatment.

Serious Adverse Events. The serious adverse events related to peginterferon that might contraindicate the use of peginterferon in re-treatment include:

- Severe neuropsychiatric symptoms
- Suicidal thoughts or actions
- Extreme flu-like symptoms
- Severe functional impairment
- Flare or development of autoimmune disease
- Serious infection
- Worsening or development of pulmonary disease
- Marked lowering of red blood cells, white blood cells, or platelets

Severe anemia is a serious adverse event related to ribavirin, boceprevir, or telaprevir that might contraindicate the use of these drugs in a re-treatment regimen. The anemia of ribavirin is worse when ribavirin is used with the alfa interferons, because alfa interferons block the bone marrow's ability to rebuild the circulating red blood cell mass. Boceprevir and telaprevir also block the bone marrow, but, in the absence of alfa interferons, the impact on the circulating red blood cell mass is minimal. Ribavirin (and possibly either boceprevir or telaprevir) could be considered in the re-treatment of a patient who has suffered severe anemia during prior therapy, as long as the re-treatment regimen is interferon-free or contains lambda, in place of alfa, interferon.

Failure Due to Viral Resistance

A common cause of treatment failure is the emergence of variants of HCV that are resistant to the administered direct-acting antiviral (DAA). Viral resistance is detected by closely assessing the response of HCV RNA to treatment. Viral resistance is likely when the HCV RNA, which had previously been undetectable, becomes detectable while continuing the DAA. Viral resistance is also likely when the HCV RNA, which had been on the decline, begins to increase.

Each DAA selects for a different set of viral variants. The viral variants that emerge during treatment with one DAA may or may not be sensitive to treatment with a different DAA.

In the case of the currently available protease inhibitors (telaprevir and boceprevir), viral variants resistant to telaprevir will also be resistant to boceprevir, and variants resistant to boceprevir, in turn, will be resistant to telaprevir. For these reasons, it is not recommended to re-treat telaprevir or boceprevir treatment failures with boceprevir or telaprevir, respectively.

POTENTIAL OPTIONS FOR RE-TREATMENT

Lambda Interferon

If your primary reason for failing a prior course of triple therapy was intolerance to interferon-alfa (all currently available interferons are alfa interferons), lambda interferon may be useful in a re-treatment regimen. Peginterferon-lambda is being studied in Phase III clinical trials. Peginterferon-lambda may have greater antiviral potency than peginterferon-alfa and, perhaps more importantly, fewer side effects. Peginterferon-lambda inhibits the bone marrow less than the alfa interferons. Why is that good? Your bone marrow produces all of your blood cells: red blood cells, white blood cells, and platelets. Compared to alfa-interferons, patients taking lambda interferon have less anemia (lowering of red blood cells), and maintain higher levels of white blood cells (the cells that fight infection) and platelets (the cells that aid clotting). The main clinical benefits of these effects could be seen as a reduced need for ribavirin dose reduction, less transfusion of red blood cells, and the decreased use of treatments to raise red blood cells (erythropoietin analogues) or white blood cells (granulocyte-colony stimulating factors). If it is FDA-approved, peginterferon-lambda might be a better tolerated interferon if you are re-treated with an interferon-containing regimen.

Triple Therapy Using More Potent Protease Inhibitors

Three protease inhibitors, danoprevir, TMC-435, and BI-201335, are beginning Phase III clinical trials as new regimens of triple therapy. Although these drugs may offer some advantages over telaprevir or boceprevir, the resistant viral variants that emerge during telaprevir or boceprevir may be the same variants that develop resistance during treatment with danoprevir, TMC-435, and BI-201335. For this reason, triple therapy with danoprevir, TMC-435, or BI-201335 and peginterferon/ribavirin may not be effective for re-treating patients who have failed a prior course of triple therapy with either telaprevir or boceprevir.

Many other protease inhibitors are proceeding down the path of clinical development. These include vaniprevir, narlaprevir, BMS-650032, GS-9256, ACH-1625, IDX-320, VX-985, and ABT-450. Many of these compounds appear very promising as potent and well-tolerated inhibitors of the HCV NS3/4A protease. However, the resistant viral variants emerging during telaprevir or boceprevir treatment may also be resistant to some of these agents.

Triple Therapy Using Direct-Acting Antivirals Other Than Protease Inhibitors

A potentially effective strategy for re-treatment of patients with viral resistance to protease inhibitors is the use of drugs from different antiviral classes. Currently, there are three main classes: protease inhibitors, NS5B polymerase inhibitors, and inhibitors of NS5A protein. Typically, resistant viral variants to one class of antivirals retain sensitivity to the other classes. If you developed resistant viral variants to telaprevir or boceprevir (both of which are protease inhibitors), those variants would likely be sensitive to inhibitors of the NS5B polymerase or the NS5A protein.

Inhibitors of NS5B Polymerase. Polymerase inhibitors target the NS5B RNA-dependent RNA polymerase of HCV, an enzyme critical for viral replication. There are two types of polymerase inhibitors: nucleoside or non-nucleoside. Nucleoside inhibitors target the active site of NS5B polymerase, and are active against most HCV genotypes. Non-nucleoside inhibitors bind at other sites of the NS5B polymerase, and also have broad activity. An increased genetic barrier to resistance is reported for the nucleoside inhibitors, while the non-nucleoside inhibitors have had significant issues with resistance and suboptimal viral suppression. Nucleoside inhibitors might be preferred over non-nucleoside inhibitors for re-treatment in order to avoid development of multi-drug resistance. The two nucleoside polymerase inhibitors with the furthest development are mericitabine and GS-7977.

- **Mericitabine (RG-7128).** The results from the JUMP-C trial indicated an SVR of 76 percent after 12 months of response-guided therapy with mericitibine-based triple therapy. Importantly, there was no evidence of the emergence of breakthrough related to viral resistance. Although the viral responses were not as potent as one would like for re-treatment, the lack of the emergence of viral resistance is encouraging in terms of the potential for use of mericitibine in re-treating prior triple therapy failures. Nonetheless, it is likely that a QUAD regimen incorporating mericitabine with a second agent would be a preferred re-treatment regimen over peginterferon/ribavirin/mericitabine (see page 146 for more information on QUAD therapy).

- **GS-7977.** The results from the PROTON trial indicated that GS-7977-based triple therapy was very potent: nearly all treatment-naïve patients with HCV genotype 1 infection demonstrated excellent virologic response. Ninety-eight percent of patients at week four of treatment had undetectable HCV RNA, their SVR at 12 months was 91 percent, and there was no evidence of viral resistance. The high potency and lack of viral resistance suggests that a triple therapy regimen incorporating GS-7977 could be effective in re-treatment for at least a sizable proportion of patients who had failed initial treatment with telaprevir or boceprevir.

Another advantage of HCV polymerase inhibitors is they may be active against non-1 HCV genotypes. Mericitabine, GS-7977, and other NS5B polymerase inhibitors have activity against non-1 HCV genotypes.

Several additional polymerase inhibitors are at various stages of clinical investigation. These include VX-222, GS-9190, PSI-7792, BI-207127, IDX-375, IDX-184, ALS-2200, ALS-2158, MK-0608, TMC-649128, PF-868554, ANA-598, VCH-759, ABT-837093, ABT-072, ABT-333, INX-189, and GSK-625433. Many of these compounds appear very promising as potent and well-tolerated inhibitors of the HCV NS5B polymerase. Non-nucleoside polymerase inhibitors, compared to nucleoside inhibitors, have a lower barrier to the development of resistant viral variants, and would be less ideal in a regimen as the only DAA with peginterferon/ribavirin. Non-nucleoside inhibitors would likely require an additional agent from another DAA class to be maximally effective in a re-treatment regimen.

Inhibitors of NS5A Protein. Daclatasvir (BMS-790052) has demonstrated potent inhibition of NS5A and HCV replication, and is being studied in a triple therapy regimen in ongoing Phase III trials. Despite its high potency, daclatasvir has a relatively low barrier to the development of resistant viral variants. To achieve maximal potency in a re-treatment regimen, it is likely that daclatasvir will need to be combined with at least one other DAA (see page 146 for more information on QUAD therapy).

Other NS5A inhibitors are in the early phases of clinical trials. These include ACH-2928, PPI-461, AZD-7295, and others. Once again, many appear promising as components of triple therapy or other combination treatments.

HCV Genotype 1a Versus 1b

HCV genotype 1b, compared to 1a, may be particularly responsive or susceptible to re-treatment. This is due to the fact that HCV genotype 1a has a lower barrier for the emergence of viral variants resistant to the protease inhibitors. This means, during treatment of a patient infected with HCV genotype 1a, resistant viral variants may emerge that compromise virologic response. This translates to a lower chance for cure with interferon-free treatment regimens in patients infected with HCV genotype 1a. Do not be alarmed if you have HCV genotype 1a infection: the rates of SVR are excellent with many of the new treatments. Yet maximizing your chances to achieve SVR if you are infected with HCV genotype 1a may require interferon.

QUAD Therapy

QUAD therapy implies the use of two direct-acting antivirals with peginterferon/ribavirin. The early experience with QUAD therapy in a very small number of patients has been promising. QUAD therapy dramatically enhances SVR, and also blocks the emergence of resistant viral variants.

Daclatasvir Plus BMS–650032 Plus Peginterferon/Ribavirin. This combination of inhibitors of NS5A and NS3/4A protease plus peginterferon/ribavirin was studied in 10 null responders to prior treatment with peginterferon/ribavirin who were infected with HCV genotype 1, mostly with subtype 1a. At least nine of the 10 patients achieved SVR, despite only 24 weeks of treatment. Given the high rate of viral response in these null responders to peginterferon/ribavirin, it is likely that this regimen may also be of benefit to patients whose prior treatment had been triple therapy with protease inhibitors.

Additional QUAD regimens are currently under study. QUAD therapy may push the limits of SVR to near 100 percent, will likely cover the broad range of genotypes and subtypes, and could even be effective in the re-treatment of failures of triple therapy. The high potency of QUAD therapy reduces the need for baseline predictors of response (such as

IL28B polymorphism), prevents the emergence of resistant viral variants, and allows further shortening of the duration of antiviral therapy.

Interferon-Free Treatment Options

As you know, the side effects of interferon and the burden of injections dominate management issues for patients and providers. Elimination of interferon could greatly simplify the re-treatment regimen, and improve patient adherence and compliance. Several interferon-free protocols are currently under clinical investigation, but none have yet been tested in triple therapy failures. Re-treatment regimens for patients with HCV genotype 1b infection may be less complicated than re-treatment regimens for HCV genotype 1a.

Daclatasvir plus BMS-650032 was given for 24 weeks to 10 Japanese null responders to prior peginterferon/ribavirin. All were infected with HCV subtype 1b, and the SVR was 100 percent (AASLD 2011). If this result holds up in trials of larger numbers of patients, it is possible that patients with HCV genotype 1b who have failed triple therapy might respond to re-treatment with interferon-free, ribavirin-free DUAL DAA therapy.

However, this same regimen, when taken as DUAL DAA therapy, was much less effective against HCV genotype 1a. In contrast, the two DAAs when taken with peginterferon/ribavirin were very effective in a small number of patients. Although many additional studies are needed, it is possible the DUAL DAA therapy might be developed for triple therapy failures with HCV genotype 1b, while QUAD regimens (likely including ribavirin, with or without interferon) will be needed for the re-treatment of HCV genotype 1a.

A number of interferon-free multi-drug regimens (including inhibitors of all three antiviral classes, with and without ribavirin) are currently under study. Many of these combinations appear promising as interferon-free regimens that could potentially be effective for re-treatment.

Another class of compounds called cyclophyllin inhibitors, which act on host mechanisms, may play a future role in re-treatment, likely as a component of a multi-drug regimen.

FIGURE 7A: EMERGING TREATMENTS
AND POTENTIAL TIMELINES

> **2014**
>> **TT – PI**   TMC 435   PR
>> **TT – PI**   BI 201335   PR
>> **IFN – Free**   PSI 7977   R (G 2/3)

> **2015**
>> **TT- NS5A-I**   BMS Daclatasvir   PR
>> **TT – NI**   PSI 7997   PR
>> **IFN – Free**   PSI 7977   R (G 1)

> **At or after 2015**
>> **QUAD**   PI/NS5A-I, PI/NI,   PR
>>   PI/NNI
>>
>> **IFN-Free**   PI/NS5A-I, PI/NI,   ± R
>>   PI/NI or NNI/NS5A-I

FIGURE 7A: Several options for future treatments and potential timelines for FDA approvals are shown. Patients failing prior treatment with peginterferon/ribavirin or current triple therapy will likely have many options for future therapy. It is highly likely that re-treatment regimens will be individualized based upon tolerability, side effects, and prior patterns of viral resistance. Abbreviations: TT, triple therapy; PI, protease inhibitor; PR, peginterferon/ribavirin; IFN, interferon; G, HCV genotype; NS5A-I, inhibitor of the NS5A protein of HCV; NI, nucleoside inhibitor of NS5B polymerase of HCV; NNI, non-nucleoside inhibitor of NS5B polymerase of HCV; QUAD, two direct acting antivirals with peginterferon/ribavirin.

CONCLUDING REMARKS

Do not despair if you fail to respond to telaprevir-based or boceprevir-based triple therapy—many options will be available in the near future to treat your hepatitis C. Options could include new interferons, more potent protease inhibitors, NS5A inhibitors, inhibitors of the NS5B polymerase, or other emerging treatments. A number of combination treatments are currently under investigation, and many have demonstrated activity and promise in treating even the most resistant forms of HCV. In this chapter, I provided some guidelines for future treatment options. Remember that none of these have yet been studied or approved by the FDA for the re-treatment of patients with HCV who failed to clear HCV with triple therapy. Nonetheless, patients should be encouraged by the rapid advances in HCV treatment and the potential plethora of new agents that could possibly be available in the future.

BIBLIOGRAPHY

1. Houghton M. Discovery of the hepatitis C virus. *Liver Int.* 2009; 29: 82–88.

2. Radetsky P. *The Invisible Invaders: Viruses and the Scientists Who Pursue Them.* Boston, MA: Little, Brown and Company; 1994: 8.

3. Houghton M. The long and winding road leading to the identification of the hepatitis C virus. *J Hepatol.* 2009; 51: 939–948.

4. Kuiken C, Simmonds P. Nomenclature and numbering of the hepatitis C virus. *Methods Mol Biol.* 2009; 510: 33–53.

5. Simmonds P, Bukh J, Combet C, et al. Consensus proposals for a unified system of nomenclature of hepatitis C virus genotypes. *Hepatology.* 2005; 42: 962–973.

6. Antaki N, Craxi A, Kamal S, et al. The neglected hepatitis C virus genotypes 4, 5 and 6: an international consensus report. *Liver Int.* 2010; 30: 342–355.

7. Tohme RA, Holmberg SD. Is sexual contact a major mode of hepatitis C virus transmission? *Hepatology.* 2010; 52: 1497–1505.

8. Ge D, Fellay J, Thompson AJ, et al. Genetic variation in IL28B predicts hepatitis C treatment-induced viral clearance. *Nature.* 2009; 461: 399–401.

9. Thomas DL, Seeff LB. Natural history of hepatitis C. *Clin Liver Dis.* 2005; 9: 383–98.

10. Pockros PJ. Drugs in development for chronic hepatitis C: a promising future. *Expert Opin Biol Ther.* 2011; 11: 1611–1622.

11. Jensen DM. A new era of hepatitis C therapy begins. *N Engl J Med.* 2011; 364: 1272–1274.

12. Carbone M, Neuberger J. Liver transplantation for hepatitis C and alcoholic liver disease. *J Transplant.* 2010; 2010: 893893. http://www.ncbi.nlm.nih.gov/pubmed/21209701. Accessed February 5, 2012.

13. Sievert W, Altraif I, Razavi HA, et al. A systematic review of hepatitis C virus epidemiology in Asia, Australia and Egypt. *Liver Int.* 2011; 31: 61–80.

14. Cornberg M, Razavi HA, Alberti A, et al. A systematic review of hepatitis C virus epidemiology in Europe, Canada and Israel. *Liver Int.* 2011; 31: 30–60.

15. Karmochkine M, Carrat F, Dos Santos O, Cacoub P, Raguin G. A case-control study of risk factors for hepatitis C infection in patients with unexplained routes of infection. *J Viral Hepat.* 2006; 13: 775–782.

16. Weusten J, Vermeulen M, van Drimmelen H, Lelie N. Refinement of a viral transmission risk model for blood donations in seroconversion window phase screened by nucleic acid testing in different pool sizes and repeat test algorithms. *Transfusion.* 2011; 51: 203–215.

17. Hakre S, Peel SA, O'Connell RJ, et al. Transfusion-transmissible viral infections among US military recipients of whole blood and

platelets during Operation Enduring Freedom and Operation Iraqi Freedom. *Transfusion*. 2011; 51: 473–485.

18. Kelen GD, Green GB, Purcell RH, et al. Hepatitis B and hepatitis C in emergency department patients. *N Engl J Med*. 1992; 326: 1399–1404.

19. Hutin Y, Hauri A, Chiarello L, et al. Best infection control practices for intradermal, subcutaneous, and intramuscular needle injections. *Bull World Health Organ*. 2003; 81: 491–500.

20. Quaranta A, Napoli C, Fasano F, Montagna C, Caggiano G, Montagna MT. Body piercing and tattoos: a survey on young adults' knowledge of the risks and practices in body art. *BMC Public Health*. 2011; 11: 774-782.

21. Haley RW, Fischer RP. Commercial tattooing as a potentially important source of hepatitis C infection. Clinical epidemiology of 626 consecutive patients unaware of their hepatitis C serologic status. *Medicine*. 2001; 80: 134–151.

22. Roy E, Haley N, Leclerc P, Boivin JF, Cédras L, Vincelette J. Risk factors for hepatitis C virus infection among street youths. *CMAJ*. 2001; 165: 557–560.

23. Indolfi G, Resti M. Perinatal transmission of hepatitis C virus infection. *J Med Virol*. 2009; 81: 836–843.

24. Nakamura I, Tanaka Y, Ochiai K, Moriyasu F, Mizokami M, Imawari M. Clarification of interspousal hepatitis C virus infection in acute hepatitis C patients by molecular evolutionary analyses: Consideration on sexual and non-sexual transmission between spouses. *Hepatol Res*. 2011; 41: 838–845.

25. Larsen C, Chaix ML, Le Strat Y, et al. Gaining Greater Insight into HCV Emergence in HIV-Infected Men Who Have Sex with Men: The HEPAIG Study. *PLoS One.* 2011; 6: 12. http://www.ncbi.nlm.nih.gov/pubmed/22216248. Accessed February 5, 2012.

26. Centers for Disease Control and Prevention (CDC). Sexual transmission of hepatitis C virus among HIV-infected men who have sex with men—New York City, 2005–2010. *MMWR.* 2011; 60: 945–950.

27. Pereira BJ, Wright TL, Schmid CH, Levey AS. A controlled study of hepatitis C transmission by organ transplantation. The New England Organ Bank Hepatitis C Study Group. *Lancet.* 1995; 345: 484–487.

28. Pereira BJ, Milford EL, Kirkman RL, et al. Prevalence of hepatitis C virus RNA in organ donors positive for hepatitis C antibody and in the recipients of their organs. *N Engl J Med.* 1992; 327: 910–915.

29. Tesi RJ, Waller K, Morgan CJ, Delaney S, et al. Transmission of hepatitis C by kidney transplantation—the risks. *Transplantation.* 1994; 57: 826–831.

30. Pereira BJ, Milford EL, Kirkman RL, Levey AS. Transmission of hepatitis C virus by organ transplantation. *N Engl J Med.* 1991; 325: 454–460.

31. Centers for Disease Control and Prevention (CDC). Transmission of hepatitis C virus through transplanted organs and tissue—Kentucky and Massachusetts, 2011. *MMWR.* 2011; 60: 1697–1700.

32. Bossler A, Gunsolly C, Pyne MT, et al. Performance of the COBAS® AmpliPrep/COBAS TaqMan® automated system for hepatitis C virus (HCV) quantification in a multi-center comparison. *J Clin Virol.* 2011; 50: 100–103.

33. Tan CH, Low SC, Thng CH. APASL and AASLD Consensus Guidelines on Imaging Diagnosis of Hepatocellular Carcinoma: A Review. *Int J Hepatol.* 2011; 2011: 519783.
http://www.ncbi.nlm.nih.gov/pubmed/22007313. Accessed February 5, 2012.

34. Rockey DC, Caldwell SH, Goodman ZD, Nelson RC, Smith AD, American Association for the Study of Liver Diseases. Liver Biopsy. *Hepatology.* 2009; 49: 1017–1044.

35. Sanyal AJ, Fontana RJ, Di Bisceglie AM, et al. The prevalence and risk factors associated with esophageal varices in subjects with hepatitis C and advanced fibrosis. *Gastrointest Endosc.* 2006; 64: 855–864.

36. Fried MW. Hepatitis C infection with normal liver chemistry tests. *Clin Gastroenterol Hepatol.* 2008; 6: 503–505.

37. Malinchoc M, Kamath PS, Gordon FD, Peine CJ, Rank J, ter Borg PC. A model to predict poor survival in patients undergoing transjugular intrahepatic portosystemic shunts. *Hepatology.* 2000; 31: 864–871.

38. Kamath PS, Wiesner RH, Malinchoc M, et al. A model to predict survival in patients with end-stage liver disease. *Hepatology.* 2001; 33: 464–470.

39. Angermayr B, Cejna M, Karnel F, et al. Child-Pugh versus MELD score in predicting survival in patients undergoing transjugular intrahepatic portosystemic shunt. *Gut.* 2003; 52: 879–885.

40. Salerno F, Merli M, Cazzaniga M, et al. MELD score is better than Child-Pugh score in predicting 3-month survival of patients undergoing transjugular intrahepatic portosystemic shunt. *J Hepatol.* 2002; 36: 494–500.

41. Wiesner R, Edwards E, Freeman R, et al. Model for end-stage liver disease (MELD) and allocation of donor livers. *Gastroenterology.* 2003; 124: 91–96.

42. Brown RS Jr, Kumar KS, Russo MW, et al. Model for end-stage liver disease and Child-Turcotte-Pugh score as predictors of pre-transplantation disease severity, posttransplantation outcome, and resource utilization in United Network for Organ Sharing status 2A patients. *Liver Transpl.* 2002; 8: 278–284.

43. Martínez SM, Crespo G, Navasa M, Forns X. Noninvasive assessment of liver fibrosis. *Hepatology.* 2011; 53: 325–335.

44. Schmeltzer PA, Talwalkar JA. Noninvasive tools to assess hepatic fibrosis: ready for prime time. *Gastroenterol Clin North Am.* 2011; 40: 507–521.

45. Sterling RK, Smith JO. Systematic review: non-invasive methods of fibrosis analysis in chronic hepatitis C. *Aliment Pharmacol Thers.* 2009; 30: 557–576.

46. Ilan Y. Review article: the assessment of liver function using breath tests. *Aliment Pharmacol Ther.* 2007; 26: 1293–1302.

47. Ilan Y. A fourth dimension in decision making in hepatology. *Hepatol Res.* 2010; 40: 1143–1154.

48. Everson GT, Martucci MA, Shiffman ML, et al. Portal-systemic shunting in patients with fibrosis or cirrhosis due to chronic hepatitis C: The minimal model for measuring cholate clearances and shunt. *Aliment Pharmacol. Ther* 2007; 26: 401–410.

49. Everson GT, Shiffman ML, Hoefs JC, et al. Quantitative liver function tests improve the prediction of clinical outcomes in chronic hepatitis C: Results from the HALT-C trial. *Hepatology.* 2011. http://www.ncbi.nlm.nih.gov/pubmed/22030902. Accessed February 5, 2012.

50. Ghany MG, Strader DB, Thomas DL, Seeff LB, American Association for the Study of Liver Diseases. Diagnosis, management, and treatment of hepatitis C: An update. *Hepatology.* 2009; 49: 1335–1374.

51. Ghany MG, Nelson DR, Strader DB, Thomas DL, Seeff LB, American Association for Study of Liver Diseases. An update on treatment of genotype 1 chronic hepatitis C virus infection: 2011 practice guideline by the American Association for the Study of Liver Diseases. *Hepatology.* 2011; 54: 1433–1444.

52. Seeff LB, Curto TM, Szabo G, et al. Herbal product use by persons enrolled in the hepatitis C Antiviral Long-Term Treatment Against Cirrhosis (HALT-C) Trial. *Hepatology.* 2008; 47: 605–612.

53. Fried MW, Shiffman ML, Reddy KR, et al. Peginterferon alfa-2a plus ribavirin for chronic hepatitis C virus infection. *N Engl J Med.* 2002; 347: 975–982.

54. Manns MP, McHutchison JG, Gordon SC, et al. Peginterferon alfa-2b plus ribavirin compared with interferon alfa-2b plus ribavirin for initial treatment of chronic hepatitis C: A randomised trial. *Lancet.* 2001; 358: 958–965.

55. Hadziyannis SJ, Sette H Jr, Morgan TR, et al. Peginterferon-alfa2a and ribavirin combination therapy in chronic hepatitis C: A randomized study of treatment duration and ribavirin dose. *Ann Intern Med.* 2004; 140: 346–355.

56. Morgan TR, Ghany MG, Kim HY, et al. Outcome of sustained virological responders with histologically advanced chronic hepatitis C. *Hepatology*. 2010; 52: 833–844.

57. Foster GR, Fried MW, Hadziyannis SJ, Messinger D, Freivogel K, Weiland O. Prediction of sustained virological response in chronic hepatitis C patients treated with peginterferon alfa-2a (40KD) and ribavirin. *Scand J Gastroenterol*. 2007; 42: 247–255.

58. O'Brien TR, Everhart JE, Morgan TR, et al. An IL28B genotype-based clinical prediction model for treatment of chronic hepatitis C. *PLoS One*. 2011; 6: 7.
http://www.ncbi.nlm.nih.gov/pubmed/21760886. Accessed February 5, 2012.

59. Conjeevaram HS, Fried MW, Jeffers LJ, et al. Peginterferon and ribavirin treatment in African American and Caucasian American patients with hepatitis C genotype 1. *Gastroenterology*. 2006; 131: 470–477.

60. Trotter J, Forman L, Kugelmas M, et al. Treatment of advanced hepatitis C with a low accelerating dosage regimen of antiviral therapy. *Hepatology*. 2005; 42: 255–262.

61. Everson GT, Hoefs JC, Seeff LB, et al. Impact of disease severity on outcome of antiviral therapy for chronic hepatitis C: Lessons from the HALT-C trial. *Hepatology*. 2006; 44: 1675–1684.

62. Carrión JA, Martínez-Bauer E, Crespo G, et al. Antiviral therapy increases the risk of bacterial infections in HCV-infected cirrhotic patients awaiting liver transplantation: A retrospective study. *J Hepatol*. 2009; 50: 719–728.

63. Forns X, García-Retortillo M, Serrano T, et al. Antiviral therapy of patients with decompensated cirrhosis to prevent recurrence of hepatitis C after liver transplantation. *J Hepatol.* 2003; 39: 389–396.

64. Forns X, Bruix J. Treating hepatitis C in patients with cirrhosis: The effort is worth it. *J Hepatol.* 2010; 52: 624–626.

65. Veldt BJ, Heathcote EJ, Wedemeyer H, et al. Sustained virologic response and clinical outcomes in patients with chronic hepatitis C and advanced fibrosis. *Ann Intern Med.* 2007; 147: 677–684.

66. Bruno S, Crosignani A, Facciotto C, et al. Sustained virologic response prevents the development of esophageal varices in compensated, Child-Pugh class A hepatitis C virus-induced cirrhosis. A 12-year prospective follow-up study. *Hepatology.* 2010; 51: 2069–2076.

67. Bacon BR, Gordon SC, Lawitz E, et al. Boceprevir for previously treated chronic HCV genotype 1 infection. *N Engl J Med.* 2011; 364: 1207–1217.

68. Poordad F, McCone J Jr, Bacon BR, et al. Boceprevir for untreated chronic HCV genotype 1 infection. *N Engl J Med.* 2011; 364: 1195–1206.

69. Sherman KE, Flamm SL, et al. Response-guided telaprevir combination treatment for hepatitis C virus infection. *N Engl J Med.* 2011; 365: 1014–24.

70. McHutchison JG, Manns MP, Terrault N, et al. Telaprevir for previously treated chronic HCV infection. *N Engl J Med.* 2011; 362: 1292–1303.

71. Jacobson IM, McHutchison JG, Dusheiko G, et al. Telaprevir for previously untreated chronic hepatitis C virus infection. *N Engl J Med.* 2011; 364: 2405–2416.

72. McHutchison JG, Gordon SC, Schiff ER, et al. Interferon alfa-2b alone or in combination with ribavirin as initial treatment for chronic hepatitis C. Hepatitis Interventional Therapy Group. *N Engl J Med*. 1998; 339: 1485–1492.

73. Davis GL, Esteban-Mur R, Rustgi V, et al. Interferon alfa-2b alone or in combination with ribavirin for the treatment of relapse of chronic hepatitis C. International Hepatitis Interventional Therapy Group. *N Engl J Med*. 1998; 339: 1493–1499.

74. Davis GL. Recombinant alfa-interferon treatment of non-A and non-B (type C) hepatitis: Review of studies and recommendations for treatment. *J Hepatol*. 1990; 11 (Suppl 1): S72-77.

75. Davis GL, Balart LA, Schiff ER, et al. Treatment of chronic hepatitis C with recombinant interferon alfa. A multicenter randomized, controlled trial. Hepatitis Interventional Therapy Group. *N Engl J Med*. 1989; 321: 1501–1506.

76. Hoofnagle JH. Course and outcome of hepatitis C. *Hepatology*. 2002; 36: 21–29.

77. Swain MG, Lai MY, Shiffman ML, et al. A sustained virologic response is durable in patients with chronic hepatitis C treated with peginterferon alfa-2a and ribavirin. *Gastroenterology*. 2010; 139: 1593–1601.

78. Pawlotsky JM. Treatment failure and resistance with direct-acting antiviral drugs against hepatitis C virus. *Hepatology*. 2011; 53: 1742–1751.

79. Hiraga N, Imamura M, Abe H, et al. Rapid emergence of telaprevir resistant hepatitis C virus strain from wildtype clone in vivo. *Hepatology*. 2011; 54: 781–788.

80. Foster GR, Hézode C, Bronowicki JP, et al. Telaprevir alone or with peginterferon and ribavirin reduces HCV RNA in patients with chronic genotype 2 but not genotype 3 infections. *Gastroenterology*. 2011; 141: 881–889.

81. Charlton M. Telaprevir, boceprevir, cytochrome P450 and immunosuppressive agents—a potentially lethal cocktail. *Hepatology*. 2011; 54: 3–5.

82. Garg V, van Heeswijk R, Lee JE, Alves K, Nadkarni P, Luo X. Effect of telaprevir on the pharmacokinetics of cyclosporine and tacrolimus. *Hepatology*. 2011; 54: 20–27.

83. Vachon ML, Dieterich DT. The HIV/HCV-coinfected patient and new treatment options. *Clin Liver Dis*. 2011; 15: 585–596.

84. Jensen DM, Pol S. IL28B genetic polymorphism testing in the era of direct acting antivirals therapy for chronic hepatitis C: Ten years too late. *Liver Int*. 2012; 32: 74–78.

85. Fried MW, Hadziyannis SJ, Shiffman ML, Messinger D, Zeuzem S. Rapid virological response is the most important predictor of sustained virological response across genotypes in patients with chronic hepatitis C virus infection. *J Hepatol*. 2011; 55: 69–75.

86. Shiffman ML, Esteban R. Triple therapy for HCV genotype 1 infection: Telaprevir or boceprevir. *Liver Int*. 2012; 32: 54–60.

87. Hézode C, Forestier N, Dusheiko G, Ferenci P, Pol S, Goeser T, Bronowicki JP, Bourlière M, Gharakhanian S, Bengtsson L, et al. Telaprevir and peginterferon with or without ribavirin for chronic HCV infection. *N Engl J Med*. 2009; 360: 1839–1850.

88. Kwo PY, Vinayek R. The therapeutic approaches for hepatitis C virus: Protease inhibitors and polymerase inhibitors. *Gut Liver.* 2011; 5: 406–417.

89. Diegelmann J, Beigel F, Zitzmann K, et al. Comparative analysis of the lambda-interferons IL-28A and IL-29 regarding their transcriptome and their antiviral properties against hepatitis C virus. *PLoS One.* 2010; 5: 12. http://www.ncbi.nlm.nih.gov/pubmed/21170333. Accessed February 5, 2012.

90. Donnelly RP, Dickensheets H, O'Brien TR. Interferon-lambda and therapy for chronic hepatitis C virus infection. *Trends Immunol.* 2011; 32: 443–450.

91. Reesink HW, Fanning GC, Farha KA, et al. Rapid HCV-RNA decline with once daily TMC435: A phase I study in healthy volunteers and hepatitis C patients. *Gastroenterology.* 2010; 138: 913–921.

92. Ciesek S, von Hahn T, Manns MP. Second-wave protease inhibitors: Choosing an heir. *Clin Liver Dis.* 2011; 15: 597–609.

93. Schlütter J. Therapeutics: New drugs hit the target. *Nature.* 2011; 474: 0–7.

94. Zeuzem S, Asselah T, Angus P, et al. Efficacy of the protease inhibitor BI 201335, polymerase inhibitor BI 207127, and ribavirin in patients with chronic HCV infection. *Gastroenterology.* 2011; 141: 2047–2055.

95. Lagacé L, White PW, Bousquet C, et al. In Vitro Resistance Profile of the Hepatitis C Virus NS3 Protease Inhibitor BI 201335. *Antimicrob Agents Chemother.* 2012; 56: 569–572.

96. Forestier N, Larrey D, Marcellin P, et al. Antiviral activity of danoprevir (ITMN-191/RG7227) in combination with pegylated interferon α-2a and ribavirin in patients with hepatitis C. *J Infect Dis*. 2011; 204: 601–608.

97. Gane EJ, Rouzier R, Stedman C, et al. Antiviral activity, safety, and pharmacokinetics of danoprevir/ritonavir plus PEG-IFN α-2a/RBV in hepatitis C patients. *J Hepatol*. 2011; 55: 972–979.

98. de Bruijne J, Bergmann JF, Reesink HW, et al. Antiviral activity of narlaprevir combined with ritonavir and pegylated interferon in chronic hepatitis C patients. *Hepatology*. 2010; 52: 1590–1599.

99. Gane EJ, Roberts SK, Stedman CA, et al. Oral combination therapy with a nucleoside polymerase inhibitor (RG7128) and danoprevir for chronic hepatitis C genotype 1 infection (INFORM-1): A randomised, double-blind, placebo-controlled, dose-escalation trial. *Lancet*. 2010; 376: 1467–1475.

100. Membreno FE, Lawitz EJ. The HCV NS5B nucleoside and non-nucleoside inhibitors. *Clin Liver Dis*. 2011; 15: 611–626.

101. Lam AM, Espiritu C, Bansal S, et al. Hepatitis C virus nucleotide inhibitors PSI-352938 and PSI-353661 exhibit a novel mechanism of resistance requiring multiple mutations within replicon RNA. *J Virol*. 2011; 85: 12334–12342.

102. Mangia A, Mottola L. What's new in HCV genotype 2 treatment. *Liver Int*. 2012; 32: 135–140.

103. Lee C. Discovery of hepatitis C virus NS5A inhibitors as a new class of anti-HCV therapy. *Arch Pharm Res*. 2011; 34: 1403–1407.

104. Chayama K, Takahashi S, Toyota J, et al. Dual therapy with the NS5A inhibitor BMS-790052 and the NS3 protease inhibitor BMS-

650032 in HCV genotype 1b-infected null responders. *Hepatology*. 2012; 55: 742-748.

105. Nettles RE, Gao M, Bifano M, et al. Multiple ascending dose study of BMS-790052, a nonstructural protein 5A replication complex inhibitor, in patients infected with hepatitis C virus genotype 1. *Hepatology*. 2011; 54: 1956–1965.

106. Lok AS, Gardiner DF, Lawitz E, et al. Preliminary study of two antiviral agents for hepatitis C genotype 1. *N Engl J Med*. 2012; 366: 216–224.

107. Watashi K. Alisporivir, a cyclosporin derivative that selectively inhibits cyclophilin, for the treatment of HCV infection. *Curr Opin Investig Drugs*. 2010; 11: 213–224.

108. Coelmont L, Hanoulle X, Chatterji U, et al. DEB025 (Alisporivir) inhibits hepatitis C virus replication by preventing a cyclophilin A induced cis-trans isomerisation in domain II of NS5A. *PLoS One*. 2010; 5: 10. http://www.ncbi.nlm.nih.gov/pubmed/21060866. Accessed February 5, 2012.

109. Patel H, Heathcote EJ. Sustained virological response with 29 days of Debio 025 monotherapy in hepatitis C virus genotype 3. *Gut*. 2011; 60: 879.

GLOSSARY

Albumin: A protein made by the liver that maintains plasma volume. Albumin levels in blood decrease when liver function worsens.

Algorithm: A diagram depicting management decisions.

ALT: Alanine aminotransferase, an enzyme specific to the liver that increases in the blood with liver injury.

Anemia: Low red blood cell count.

Ascites: Fluid buildup in the abdominal space. One cause is cirrhosis of the liver.

AST: Aspartate aminotransferase, an enzyme found in liver and other tissues that increases in the blood with liver injury.

Bilirubin: The pigment in blood, derived from the breakdown of red blood cell hemoglobin, which increases when liver function is impaired.

Cirrhosis: Extreme buildup of fibrosis in the liver leading to abnormal liver function and altered liver blood flow.

Edema: Fluid buildup in the body's tissues, most commonly in the lower extremities and ankles.

Encephalopathy: Change in mental status related to underlying liver disease.

eRVR (or eRVR'): Extended rapid virologic response. Defined as undetectable HCV RNA at treatment weeks four and 12 of telaprevir-based triple therapy (eRVR), or weeks eight and 20 of boceprevir-based triple therapy (eRVR'). Patients with eRVR stop at treatment week 24 and patients with eRVR stop at treatment week 28.

Fibrosis: Buildup of the scar tissue protein, collagen.

HCV: Hepatitis C virus.

HCV genotypes: Genetic subtypes of HCV. HCV genotypes are 1 through 6.

HCV RNA: Hepatitis C virus ribonucleic acid. Measuring HCV RNA is a way to quantify HCV. HCV RNA is measured by polymerase chain reaction assay.

IL28b Polymorphism: A genetic factor in humans that predicts one's response to interferon.

INCIVEK®: Registered tradename for telaprevir.

INR: International normalized ratio. A measure of the liver's clotting proteins that increases with hepatic impairment.

Leucopenia: Low white blood cell count.

MELD: Model for end-stage liver disease that predicts 90-day survival in patients with cirrhosis.

Null responder: A patient who experiences lack of decrease in HCV RNA by $2\log_{10}$ during prior treatment.

Partial responder: A patient who experiences a drop in HCV RNA by $2\log_{10}$ or more, but with persistently positive HCV RNA during prior treatment.

Relapse: Undetectable HCV RNA at the end of prior treatment, but return of positive HCV RNA in follow-up after treatment discontinuation.

Stop guidelines: HCV RNA levels that dictate discontinuation of treatment.

SVR: Sustained virologic response. Defined as undetectable HCV RNA at six months after the end of treatment.

Thrombocytopenia: Low platelet count.

Treatment-experienced: A patient who has had prior therapy with peginterferon/ribavirin.

Treatment-naïve: A patient who has had no prior treatment of HCV.

Triple therapy: A treatment using peginterferon and ribavirin plus telaprevir or boceprevir.

Varices: Large veins that develop in the esophagus or stomach due to portal hypertension, typically from underlying liver disease.

VICTRELIS®: Registered tradename for boceprevir.

INDEX